The All Day
Energy Diet

About the author

～ゔ～

Kathryn Marsden is well known as the author of best-selling titles such as *The Food Combining Diet*, *Food Combining in 30 Days*, and *Super Skin*. Her writings are now famous around the world and, to date, have been translated into ten languages including Chinese, Hebrew, and Spanish.

Kathryn is noted for her informative and entertaining seminars on health and fitness and her light-hearted, humorous presentations. She writes regular nutrition columns for the country's leading pharmacy publications and contributes to several top women's magazines. She lives in deepest Wiltshire.

KATHRYN MARSDEN

The All Day Energy Diet

PAN BOOKS

First published 1997 by Pan Books

an imprint of Macmillan Publishers Ltd
25 Eccleston Place, London, SW1W 9NF
and Basingstoke

Associated companies throughout the world

ISBN 0 330 35367 5

Copyright © Kathryn Marsden 1997

The right of Kathryn Marsden to be identified as the
author of this work has been asserted by her in accordance
with the Copyright, Designs and Patents Act 1988.

All rights reserved. No part of this publication may be
reproduced, stored in or introduced into a retrieval system, or
transmitted, in any form, or by any means (electronic, mechanical,
photocopying, recording or otherwise) without the prior written
permission of the publisher. Any person who does any unauthorized
act in relation to this publication may be liable to criminal
prosecution and civil claims for damages.

1 3 5 7 9 8 6 4 2

A CIP catalogue record for this book is available from
the British Library

Typeset by SX Composing DTP, Rayleigh, Essex
Printed and bound in Great Britain by
Mackays of Chatham plc, Chatham, Kent

This book is sold subject to the condition that it shall not,
by way of trade or otherwise, be lent, re-sold, hired out,
or otherwise circulated without the publisher's prior consent
in any form of binding or cover other than that in which
it is published and without a similar condition including this
condition being imposed on the subsequent purchaser.

For Richard

Contents

☙

Foreword by Dr John Briffa

࿇

I remember when I first took an interest in the subject of nutrition. Having become disillusioned with some aspects of conventional medicine quite soon after qualifying as a doctor, I felt enormous enthusiasm for the possibility that good food might be used therapeutically to improve health. I was eager to learn but also ignorant. During my six years of medical training, I received no worthwhile tuition on the subject of diet and so had no idea where to find the information I was looking for.

Starting in the health section of a local bookshop, I browsed avidly and bought nutrition books on a regular basis. There was certainly no shortage of information out there but making sense of it proved more difficult than I had anticipated. Many publications contained either no explanation for the advice they offered or made the biochemistry texts I had studied at medical school seem like child's play! If a health book contained recipes, I often felt the need for a cordon bleu cookery course to enable me to follow them. As a result, many of those that I bought in the early days were shelved after the first or second chapter and, to this day, remain unread.

It was on one of my book browsing sessions that I came across a title by Kathryn Marsden called *The Food Combining Diet*. An instant best-seller and now a classic, this easy-to-follow paperback made complete sense of what I had believed, until then, to be a complex and unworkable form of eating. What's more, the recipes were within the grasp of even my limited culinary skills!

Now, as a practising Nutritional Physician, I continue to read all Kathryn's books with equal enthusiasm. Her writings are always clear, easy to follow and come liberally seasoned with common sense and essential humour. In *The All Day Energy Diet*, she tackles the most familiar complaints of all; fatigue, lack of vitality and weight problems. This book is packed with readable information designed to put more pep into anybody's life. Follow its advice and you cannot fail to feel the difference in your energy levels and general well-being.

Dr John Briffa BSc(Hons), MB BS(Lond)
Nutritional Physician

Preamble

࿇

Ever get the sneakiest sense that your life is there for everyone else's benefit? Let me guess!

- You never have time to yourself?
- Every day is so frantic that you are permanently
  exhausted? Or you're uptight and can't concentrate?
- Your co-ordination is terrible?
- Your mood flip-flops wearily between grumpy and
  sleepy? Or you've felt grotty for so long that feeling
  great is a forgotten dream?
- Or, perhaps, you've never been happy about your hips,
  thighs, or bloated tum, rotund rear or portly paunch but
  you just can't be bothered to go another round with the
  low-fat rubber cheese and fresh-air crackers? Anyway, it
  didn't make much difference when you did.
- Or maybe you're tired all the time?

Man or woman, younger or older, if you're one of the thou-
sands of people who suffer from tiredness syndrome, be comforted by the fact that you're not alone. Many practitioners
now agree that, in the vast majority of cases, this kind of
exhaustion can be linked very firmly to diet. Intolerance to
certain foods, poor digestion, bowel problems, low blood
sugar and incorrect dieting are key factors.

If any of this sounds like you, then The All Day Energy

Diet could be just the tonic you need.

- Designed as an exhausted person's easygoing guide to renewed vigour.
- Packed with top tips on the best way to balance your weight, lift lethargy, and rediscover that lost vitality.
- Advice on how to beat brain fatigue, improve mood, and beat 'the blues'.
- And on how to keep that all-important blood glucose in balance.
- All gathered from practitioner experience, patient case histories, and up-to-date research.
- There are even some fun suggestions to nourish your love life.

plus

- Effective nutritional support if you really want to give up smoking but, until now, have been afraid of swapping cigarettes for spare tyres!

The All Day Energy Diet explains why some foods can cause fatigue and how others can revive and restore. If you've been a bit under par of late, use The All Day Energy Eating Plan to help hasten recovery. Learn about the importance of certain vitamins and minerals and catch up with the latest research into special supplements that are able to boost energy, improve concentration, and help keep weight in normal balance.

It's been estimated that as many as fifty in every hundred people don't absorb nourishment from their food supply well enough to maintain optimum health and energy. But the reasons shouldn't surprise us. We work long hours, get less than adequate sleep, eat a skimpy breakfast or forget it altogether, miss meals during the day because we haven't had time to stop or shop, fill up on less-than-healthy snacks, and rely too often on take-aways and convenience meals because we're too exhausted to prepare food from scratch. But, to maintain steady supplies of energy, we need regular pit-stops for quality fuel. Without them, the level of glucose in our blood drops and our stamina slumps accordingly.

Let's face it, most of us know the difference between eating healthily and unhealthily, but I bet the majority would probably admit that we only really look at food from the perspective of whether or not the family will eat it or how long it takes to prepare! We might fret a bit about the fat content but otherwise tend to ignore our own nutritional needs and preferences. What about how we digest our food, what we mix with what, how much we eat at one sitting, or the times of day we choose to eat? Did you know that any and all of these factors can have a profound effect on our health? After ten years as a nutritionist seeing patients in a busy clinic, I have witnessed endless examples of how certain foods aggravate existing illnesses, how others can encourage better health and a few that have some pretty special healing properties! Clinical experience certainly demonstrates that managing the diet a little more carefully can contribute to a reduction of symptoms and encourage the body to function more efficiently and energetically.

The Catch 22 is that we often have good reason for not eating as well as we should. Sometimes certain foods just don't agree with us. Avoiding them may help to reduce symptoms (such as bloating, irritable bowel, or migraine, for example) but this also means we risk giving up too much and restricting the variety in our diets and, along with it, the nutrients we need to maintain energy levels. We may worry that eating full meals encourages us to pile on the pounds. But did you know that, in some cases, food *intolerance* can be the sole cause of weight problems, irrespective of how much we eat?

If you're worried about your weight, forget the dreaded 'D' word and take a new direction. Dismiss deprivation dieting – as in 'low fat, tastes foul, always famished'. The 'Diet' in the All Day Energy title is all about balance and flexibility, helping you towards improved health and balanced weight control. No starvation, no suffering, and definitely no slop-in-a-cup diet drinks! If you're having a podgy day, your zip is stuck, your waistband is wedged, or you're completely knackered, what you need is genuine help and advice that really works. The last thing you want is a dictatorial tome full of high-handed, impossible to follow theories on how it's all your fault for not eating right in the first place. You know the kind of thing.

The inference is always the same. You're overweight because you eat too much. The only way to lose it is to eat less but you're defeated before you begin because you've already cut back to practically nothing. No wonder you're worn out!

But it isn't your fault. Dieting regimes that rely on drastic calorie reduction are *bound* to make you tired because they aren't able to provide you with enough energy-producing nutrients for your daily needs. In addition to which, they work only while you're following them, leaving you high, dry, and hungry at the end of it all. If calorie counting brought successful long-term results, why is it that everyone you know is always on a diet?

Ironically, eating a *high* calorie diet doesn't necessarily make a person energetic either. The body isn't designed to take large amounts of food on board at one time. Eating too much causes blood to be diverted from other parts of the body (including the brain and the muscles) to the digestive system to help deal with the overload of food. Result? Loss of energy and a feeling of lethargy. Eating smaller amounts *more often* allows the digestion to work more efficiently without putting undue strain on the rest of the system. But that doesn't mean that All Day Energy meals are frugal. Far from it. As you'll see from the recipes, the meal choices are designed to give you energy just when you need it.

The All Day Energy Eating Plan takes care of your health by providing the right levels of dietary fibre and making sure you have enough fresh vegetables and fruit without you having to give it a thought. But it also recognizes the importance of treats and indulgences. To help you make the healthiest choices, Getting Started (Chapter 7) guides you towards the really good for you foods and, at the same time, steers you gently away from common allergens and from items that are not so nutritious.

Better still, on The All Day Energy Diet, you don't have to give up those treats that you really enjoy. For example, if you truly crave a large chocolate-laden cappuccino and gooey pastry, then, expert advice confirms, there is good reason to go for it. Music to the ears of that one-third of the nation's female population who apparently prefer chocolate to sex.

OK. So there are advantages. You can GET chocolate.

But did you know that lack of interest in sex can be related to diet too? Not only can food be the music of love but what you eat at dinner could make a delicious difference to your dynamism, performance, and fulfilment. On the other hand, choosing the wrong foods could leave you slipping into the arms of Morpheus instead of the arms of your loved one. If you (or your partner) have been more

interested lately in snoozing than in sensual sex, read on;
The All Day Energy Diet could give you all-night energy
too. For gourmet sex you need special nourishment. Try
some of the finger-licking recipes in Part 4 and the Tasty
Titbits in Chapter 5.

Throughout The All Day Energy Eating Plan, you'll find
a whole host of tasty alternatives to those things you imag-
ined you'd have to say goodbye to forever. For example, if
chips take your fancy (whose don't they?), forgo the low-fibre
fat-laden kind and indulge your hankering by choosing the
healthy and delicious version on page 158.

An All Day Energy *priority* is that, as well as being health-
giving, *eating should be agreeable and appetising*. After all, it's a
social activity, something to be enjoyed not dreaded. The
trouble is, we've become so obsessed with the ideas that anything flavourful and filling is bound to be bad for the heart
but that if it tastes terrible it must be good for the bowels –
we've lost the ability to relax and take pleasure from mealtimes.

Look at the way we handle dieting resolutions, especially
those good intentions that manifest themselves just after
Christmas. The New Year should be a time for enjoyable
anticipation, positive thinking, and personal growth, and yet
we're swamped with pressure to give things up. And it's all
emotional blackmail based on the threat that 'if you don't do
this your health will suffer'. The first day of January is one
often overloaded with guilt about the effects of festive indulgences. The rest of the month is a miserable hotchpotch of
hunger, cravings, and niggardly recipes that are supposed to
be something special just because they can boast 'only six
calories per serving'. No wonder we are stressed and
depressed.

Psychologists researching the effects of denial on our health have found that *everyday pleasures contribute important benefits to our long-term well-being*. There is clear scientific data to show that 'spoiling ourselves' can make us feel calmer and more relaxed whereas denial does the opposite. Medical evidence has established that happy people live longer. Since the life we have is the only one we are living, enjoying it to the full seems like a sensible move!

Changing the way we eat bestows many other health benefits, too. Good grub can help to beat the blues, improve mood and attitude, enhance concentration, and boost brain power. No, not a spurious claim; a scientific fact. Food, say the experts, can have a far-reaching effect on memory and alertness as well as on energy levels and bodyweight.

All the recipes that appear in The All Day Energy Diet are all 'home-grown'; in other words, tried and tested many times in my own kitchen and on willing family, friends, and former patients. The criteria were that:

- All the meals should be quick and easy to prepare from ingredients that are readily available;
- Meals should be satisfying and nutritious, filling but not fattening, avoiding the common allergens that are known to aggravate bloating and weight problems;
- Recipes should be flexible (they won't fall apart if you leave out one particular ingredient or substitute another);
- Meals need to be interchangeable, i.e. lunches for dinners, snacks for suppers, etc.;
- Menus must take into account that most working people have limited amounts of time available for time-

consuming recipes and have little choice but to rely on at
least some convenience foods;
* Menus must be healthy as well as interesting;
* For those who don't eat meat, there should be fish dishes
  and vegetarian options;
* And because I know just what it's like when you need a
  meal in a hurry – or don't always have time to shop for
  individual items – I've included a few time-saving
  shortcuts.

As you will see from the fresh produce suggestions in Chapter 7,
The All Day Energy Plan encourages a greater variety of ingredients. Any time you're stuck for ideas, turn to these pages before
you write your shopping list.

As you wend your way through the recipe section, you'll
see that the instructions as to portion sizes are not carved in
stone. This is deliberate. Restricting someone to two ounces
of this or twenty grams of that is akin to calorie regulation
and limitation. Most people are able to judge whether they
need small or large portions at a particular meal. The All Day
Energy Eating Plan respects this inner intelligence, encouraging you to enjoy regular meals (including snacks if you feel
you need them) and to eat until you are comfortably full.

The old adage about finishing a meal and feeling that you
always have room for another mouthful is a useful one to follow. This way, your appetite will be satisfied naturally. If you
end a meal feeling stuffed to overflowing or bloated and
unable to move, then you know and I know that the extra
food will probably end up being stored as FAT!

If you've had your fill of rabbit food regimes or if every

mealtime seems like nothing more than a maths lesson, it's time to look at food from a different perspective! Over the next few weeks, The All Day Energy Diet will show you how to:

- Give your system a well-deserved rest
- Identify troublesome foods
- Break the lethargy barrier
- Beat the bloat
- Boost 'brain power'
- Sustain your stamina throughout the day
- Help you to find your natural weight

and

- Leave you with a renewed feeling of well-being.

None of the advice is difficult to follow and – big bonus – it may even improve your sex life.

Go for it now and feel great!

Wishing you health and happiness.

Kathryn Marsden
Wiltshire, England

If You Do Nothing Else . . .

๛

- Drink more water. Have supplies everywhere. By the bed, in the kitchen, around the house, at work. Take a mouthful every time you pass by and you'll soon increase your fluid intake to healthier levels. Great for the skin and can be especially helpful if you suffer with bloating, constipation or an irritable bladder or bowel.
- Breathe more deeply. Yawning and stretching is a good way to push more oxygen around the body.
- Every hour or so throughout the day, think 'shoulders'. You'll probably find that they are hunched and tense. Relax them.
- Every now and then, walk away from the task in hand and take a five-minute break.
- Empty your bladder more often. Most of us have a habit of 'putting off' visits to the bathroom on the basis that we're too busy but you'll be amazed at how bladder pressure can disturb energy levels and concentration.
- Take a brisk walk in the fresh air – every day if you can, but at least three times a week. Exercise increases energy, lifts mood and helps fight the flab.
- Laugh more and take life a little less seriously. Sending 'smile' messages to your cells really does improve well-being.

- Get plenty of sleep. Sounds simplistic but is fundamental to good health.
- Wake up to breakfast. Eating regular meals helps to keep blood glucose and cholesterol stable, enhances concentration and keeps energy levels high. And, believe it or not, grazing 'little and often' is best for balancing bodyweight, too.
- Read the section 'GETTING STARTED' on page 107. Mug up on the foods that really are good for you and try to cut back on those that we know are not so helpful.
- Eat more fresh fruit – between meals is best.
- Try to make vegetables a *main* ingredient of your main meals, not just a garnish or side dish.
- Never follow extreme or excessive eating habits, very low calorie diets or overly restricted regimes.
- Treat yourself to a favourite meal or snack once a week whether it's supposed to be nutritious or not – and enjoy it thoroughly.
- With either breakfast or lunch every day, take a multivitamin/mineral supplement. Buy the best quality that you can afford. (See Resources on page 185 for advice).

PART ONE

Losing Weight The All Day Energy Way

ONE

The weigh you want to be

৵

TOP TIPS FOR SUCCESSFUL DIETING
WHY COUNTING CALORIES CAN BE BAD FOR YOUR HEALTH
THE REAL FACTS ABOUT FAT AND CHOLESTEROL
HOW TO COPE IF YOU SMOKE
EXERCISING COMMON SENSE

৵

'Never eat more than you can lift.'
Miss Piggy

If your weight is getting you down because you can't keep it down, or if you've had enough deprivation dieting to last you a lifetime, then read on. If you're confused about cholesterol, flummoxed by fat, or if you feel that your entire life has become a permanent 'calorie-controlled diet', then stay with me. OK, we all know that a diet overloaded with fatty foods, rich sauces and tempting gateaux will pile on the pounds but that doesn't mean it's necessary to give up and suffer. There are easier, healthier ways to keep fit than counting and cutting kilojoules or enduring boring fat-free convenience food!

At one time or another, most of us have made the effort to yield that extra baggage by reducing our intake. After all, it's well known that excess weight is caused by eating too much and exercising too little! Or, as dieticians and doctors like to put it, 'obesity develops when the number of calories consumed exceeds the amount expended'.

But does it? Well, that's the generally accepted wisdom. So it's interesting that, in all my years in nutritional practice, I found only occasional instances where overweight was caused by overeating. And of the many patients I have seen, only a handful were helped long term by fat reduction or calorie restriction. As a result, I've become increasingly disillusioned with the reduce calories/reduce fat approach.

But the official view reigns supreme. I'm sure you've noticed it; the underlying but implicit assumption that the majority of plumper people could be lean and lithe if only they would pull themselves together, get into some decent eating habits and work off a few litres of sweat at the gym.

Although diet and exercise do play a definite and worthwhile role in maintaining balanced body weight, there is, in fact, mounting evidence to show that obesity is far more likely to be linked to a disordered metabolism. In other words, spare tyres and love handles may have more to do with an individual's biochemistry, physiology, and heredity than with how much food they consume.

In my experience in clinical practice, the majority of overweights were linked to food intolerance, poor digestion, candidiasis, vitamin/mineral deficiencies, hypoglycaemia and cravings, wayward hormones, or a combination of these problems. Removing a handful of common allergens, improving digestive function, and upgrading nutrient intake has resulted in healthy weight loss and better water balance.

Small changes to a normal diet are often all that are needed!

This is a comforting thought indeed for all those dedicated souls who have spent years trying to brainwash themselves, unsuccessfully, that air-filled bread and polyunsaturated axle grease are actually good for them.

It is sad, though, that anything other than weird weight loss programmes or curious crash diets are not usually considered sufficiently sensational or attention grabbing to make the headlines. Which means that most people stick to them like superglue even if they never achieve long-term success, simply because they think they are doing the right thing.

When it comes to good health and sustained energy, I have seen far more success where the principles laid out in The All Day Energy Diet have been put into practice. Ingredients are wholesome and easy to find; meals are nourishing and quick-to-prepare; yet, weight is lost without a calorie or a fat gram being counted.

To keep on promoting the view that obesity exists only as a result of overindulgence and/or idleness suggests that overweight people are somehow second-class citizens who are fat through inertia and greed. This view is unreasonable, unfair, and absolutely not true. Losing weight has become a miserable and difficult enough pastime without adding to it the pressure of guilt, blame, and failure.

It's no wonder that the well-padded suffer social stigma. Some live lives of misery, fearful of being rejected, and often turned down for jobs, being seen as lazy, slothful, and lacking in willpower. Some doctors have been known to refuse to treat overweight patients, laying the blame for the condition squarely at the door of the sufferer.

But gaining weight is not a disease, nor is it a fault of personality.

If we are to succeed, attitudes have to change. And the

unshakeable belief in counting calories and fat grams must be questioned.

Most of those who suffer with weight problems make continual efforts to shed unwanted pounds, only to find themselves caught up in the eternal yo-yo of losing weight by cutting food intake only to put it all back on again next time they glance in the direction of a chocolate bar or a burger and fries.

For women who have become victims of this very vicious circle, there is another injustice to face; an irony of nature is that males lose weight far more quickly and easily than females – due entirely (wouldn't you just know it) to their different balance of hormones. And yet ... (just a thought) ... perhaps we should ask ourselves how this equates with the fact that, despite having more body fat, women live longer than men!

Is calorie counting really necessary?

If we are going to have any chance of eradicating weight problems and the terrible tiredness that goes with them, we have to alter our outlook towards food and stop confusing quantity with quality. I know it's not easy to change the habits of a lifetime, especially if it means going against the dieting doctrine of the day. If a wart-free telly doc decrees that cutting calories is the only route to take, or a professor of nutrition with a book to sell says that all other diet books are a waste of time, it can be difficult for a failed dieter to disagree. And, on the basis that trial and tribulation equate with ultimate triumph, the martyr in us probably thinks that the only way to lose weight successfully must be to deprive ourselves of enjoyment.

So where do we go from here?

Let's say you have decided absolutely that your new diet begins tomorrow, you intend to affirm the best of eating habits for the rest of your life, and you're done with being fat forever? There's just one little problem. You've already tried every diet going and, anyway, you're too tired to be bothered.

First up, the All Day Energy Eating Plan approaches weight loss from an entirely different perspective that encourages not only healthy eating but healthy enjoyment. It avoids common food allergens but there are no long lists of taboo foods.

Secondly, don't feel bad about feeling tired. You have good reason. It's a fact that weight problems can have a significant effect upon energy levels. If you're lugging around an extra 10kg, for example, you are likely to feel fatigued. Just try walking a few yards carrying a 10kg sack of potatoes and see how quickly you run out of steam. And then try walking it while you're trying to keep to a reduced calorie diet which is giving you only about enough energy to lift a feather pillow.

You need nourishing!

Apart from being an extremely boring pastime (boredom is an energy killer anyway), a major disadvantage of calorie-restricted diets is that, by their very nature, they often restrict nutrients too.

Look at it this way. If the quantity of food is cut, the number of vitamins and minerals available that are needed to assist energy production will also be less. In the very short-term, this may not be a problem. The body will adjust and cope. However, in the longer term (and most diets run for a month or more), general health can be affected. Deciding how to lose weight without suffering from lethargy and fatigue is a common conundrum for all those hell-bent on beating the bulge.

Did you know that the old talk about stomachs shrinking if you eat less isn't true. When its empty, the stomach is only about the size of a large grapefruit and can't actually shrink. What happens is that when food intake is restricted for long periods, the stomach wall loses its elasticity, a fact which is supposed to make dieters feel full on less food. Oh yeah?

Nature decrees that, allowing for age, sex, body mass, and activity level, Mr or Mrs Average Human Being needs around 1,800 to 2,000 calories (that's approximately 7,200 to 8,000 kilojoules) per day to provide sufficient energy and nourishment for good health. But most diet programmes suggest such a low calorie level (perhaps as little as 1,000 to 1,200) that you end up wondering what happened to the main course. Shrinking food intake to two-thirds or one-half of normal might seem like a sensible idea, but do it for too long and it's perfectly possible to become malnourished. Even if you are stoical enough to stick to the wretched regime, it's probable that your weight will whizz up again once the diet is ended.

And have you noticed that no one ever tells you what to do next? The only post-diet 'after sales service' advice that the majority of diet books or fitness gurus can come up with is to increase fruits and vegetables and reduce fat intake. It didn't work; it doesn't work!

Dieting can make you rich! How about the New York housewife who, back in 1961, started a small support group to help disillusioned dieters. By 1978, she was able to sell Weight Watchers for around $100 million.

Dieting can make you fat – and fed up!

If you didn't make it to the end of the first miserable week of your 'Diet to end all diets', don't blame yourself. It doesn't mean you were weak-willed. If you've plodded patiently through a freezer full of fat-free, sugar-free, salt-free, cholesterol-free, calorie-free, taste-free pseudo food, coming out at the other end is a bit like reaching an oasis in the desert. You've been deprived of decent victuals for so long; you're desperately hungry and in need of urgent sustenance – any sustenance, just as long as it's filling and has real flavour. For goodness' sake, how can anyone in your position be expected to walk past the patisserie without stopping and savouring?

What's happening here is that, during slimming, the body is panicked into thinking it's being starved (well, it is) and tries to conserve energy by burning off fewer calories. The 'engine' slows from fast burn to an idling speed. All fine and dandy until the diet comes to an end and calorie intake goes up again. For a while, the system may still try to hold on to that energy. Weight increases because you're not burning calories; your only solution is to roll into the next diet – and the next – and, all the while, it's getting harder to get away from those creeping kilos. Proof positive, if proof were needed, that dieting can make you fat!

Dieting cycles are difficult to break and, although the results of one American study now say that frequent fluctuations in weight are not dangerous, most experts are of the view that yo-yo dieting ('doing an Oprah') probably increases the risk of heart disease, gall-bladder problems, hormone imbalances, and strokes ...

... and stressed!

Eating is generally regarded as one of life's great pleasures but dieting can be incredibly stressful. If you're following a programme that is stringent, time-consuming, depriving, not enjoyable, or in any way difficult to follow, then it is probably too stressful to be good for you.

Happily, there are far simpler ways of achieving (and maintaining) a balanced body shape than divesting yourself of cream cakes, crisps, or chocolate. Nor is there any need to feel fatigued or hungry! The All Day Energy Diet actually approves of delicious indulgences and encourages full portion sizes!

If you're worried about that bit of a paunch, podgy abdomen, or developing love handles, don't panic. It's only in Western society that these little extras are viewed as social stigmas. Orientals nurture their tums and see them as an indication of inner calm, endurance and peace of mind and body. They also believe the 'chest out, belly in' strait-jacket type of person is more prone to nervousness, tension, stress and anger and less able to express their emotions. Remind you of anyone?

So is fat the real villain?

- Fat is bad for us. It makes us ... er ... fat.
- But fat is good for us. It's an essential body nutrient.

- Fat fills us up.
- But fat causes heart disease.

- Fat keeps us warm.
- But fat clogs up the arteries.

- Fat gives us energy.
- But fat slows us down.

So much contradiction! No wonder we're confused.

So which is right?

Experts who study the relationship between nutrition and dietary fats are now suggesting that it may have been premature to recommend very low-fat diets. A point that my own nutrition tutors were making a decade ago. Too little fat, it seems, can be as dangerous as too much. But it's no good going for just any old kind. Choosing the right type and quality is vital to good health so, with this in mind, The All Day Energy Diet recipes provide a sensible and balanced intake of the healthiest fats and oils.

Fat may be good for the vocal cords. It was *Tenore pauncho* Luciano Pavarotti who is supposed to have uttered the immortal edict 'Fat people are happy because their nerves are well protected.'

It's certainly true that essential fatty acids (EFAs), special vitamin-like substances found in some fatty foods, are absolutely vital nourishment for every cell in the body and that dedicated dieters can cause themselves serious deficiencies by taking fat avoidance to extremes. In fact, certain types of low-fat diets that rely heavily on processed and packaged products are being seen as far more hazardous than eating healthier unprocessed foods that are naturally higher in fat but also rich in the protective nutrients called antioxidants as well as in dietary fibre.

Dieting can be dangerous. Allergies, behavioural problems, dry skin, eczema, splitting nails, joint stiffness, digestive disorders, cardiovascular disease, persistent infections, fluid retention, exacerbated arthritis, and sexual problems including impotence and vaginal dryness are all common symptoms of low-fat dieting. So, too, is mental, physical, and emotional exhaustion.

So is fat public enemy number one or not?

Anyone who has read any of my previous books will know that I have never advocated low-fat diets. I've seen too many patients who, as a result of going overboard on fat restriction, have created a whole pile of problems related to fat deficiency. Unfortunately, because fat is so often seen as an 'F' word ('F' for fear, I guess), low-fat foods have become big, big business.

Mention the phrase 'low-fat diet' and most people will think of a whole range of fat-reduced or fat-free processed food, e.g. low-calorie ready-meals, low-fat mayonnaise, fat-free dressing, non-fat cream, low-fat yoghurt, low-fat cheese, low-fat ice-cream, low-fat milk, low-fat fromage frais and, of course, low-fat *fat*. In other words, junk. Almost everyone I've ever met has a refrigerator full of this synthetic slop, stored in the mistaken belief that they are helping themselves towards better health. And yet, we still crave it. Fat, that is. Here's why.

- Fat is what makes food feel good and taste good.
- Fat gives food its structure; in other words, sticks it together. That's why so many fat-reduced foods are watery.
- Without fat, food falls apart, tastes terrible and is decidedly unsatisfying.
- Fat satiates the appetite and makes us feel full for longer.

Low-fat foods, on the other hand, pass through the digestive system more speedily, so you feel hungry faster. The whole thing is a confidence trick.

And then there is the margarine!

Heavily processed yellow yuck, made from something resembling engine oil, heat-treated using a very questionable process called hydrogenation and, in many instances, glued together with emulsifiers, stabilizers, colourings, and flavourings to replace the structure and flavour originally provided by the natural fat content. If you doubt this disgusting habit, plan a day trip to your local supermarket and compare the ingredients on a pack of butter with those on a low-fat spread. Or a full-fat soft cheese with a low-fat one. Take an armchair and a book on biochemistry.

You want to know how they make margarine? You might end up wishing you hadn't asked. Most commercially produced spreads start life as polyunsaturated (liquid) oils that are extracted from a variety of vegetable sources, i.e. corn, sunflower, peanut, etc. After cleaning, steaming and pressing under heat, chemical solvents are then used to increase the amount of oil extracted. The resulting liquid passes through a filter, is degummed, neutralized, washed, bleached and deodorized. To make the oil into spreadable fat, it goes through a process called hydrogenation, which chemically alters some of the polyunsaturates (liquids) into saturates (solids). Unfortunately, this process also changes beneficial 'cis' fatty acids into not-so-desirable 'trans' fatty acids which, some scientists now believe, may contribute to heart disease and clogged arteries.

I know what you're thinking. *You gave up butter for this!* The good news is that it's possible to make natural margarines without producing dangerous trans fat and without the need for solvents or hydrogenation. The method, called cold-pressing, is used to extract best quality oils. The spreads produced in this way (and available in most health-food stores and some delicatessens) cost more but are considered by many nutrition experts to be far healthier than the hydrogenated margarines available in supermarkets.

Margarine-type spreads are not the only place we find hydrogenated vegetable oils. They turn up in a whole range of packaged and processed foods. Nutrition expert Dr Udo Erasmus (*Fats That Heal, Fats That Kill,* Alive Books) goes as far as recommending that any food label that carries the 'h' word (i.e. hydrogenated) should go in the bin not the shopping basket!

Faking it!

Now, horror of horrors, we have fake fat, fat-free fat and, even, genetically engineered lean meat, good for us we are told because it's lower in fat.

You are probably getting the message that I'm not a fan of fat fiddling.

You'd be right.

How can any of it be good for our long-term health? Or for our weight? Or for our energy levels?

This is a concern I've been expressing at lectures, in classes, and in books, journals, and feature articles for a very long time. And although the vast majority of feedback has shown similar disquiet, I've been castigated and chastised by a handful of 'authorities' who saw my stance as irresponsible; so entrenched has been the official feeling that fat is hazardous in all its forms.

Now the tide is turning.

New studies are examining old findings

For a start, cholesterol (which has been tied so firmly to the fat argument) is no longer regarded as the only risk factor for heart disease. It may not be a factor at all. Some scientists are re-examining the role of saturated fat and wondering if we should ever have worried about it in the first place. Extensive research into protective nutrients known as antioxidants suggests that what happens to fat when it oxidizes (degenerates) is probably far more hazardous than the quantity of fat itself.

On top of all that, earlier advice about polyunsaturates is being reassessed. After years of promoting polys as the way to a healthy heart, manufacturers have found themselves in a right old quandary now that new research has questioned the safety of the hydrogenation process used to make spreads. Having spent several years making reassuring noises that the practice was safe and that we should have no truck with talk about the dangers of *trans fatty acids*, producers are now coming up with comforting little lines like 'low in trans fatty acids'. What they never admit is that it's perfectly possible to produce margarine without hydrogenation. There are also plenty of natural food sources where we can find uncontaminated polyunsaturated fatty acids that are extremely good for us (see page 63).

Do more artificial additives equal improved flavour?

Degrading and adulterating natural ingredients into tasteless trash is big business. If food was left as near to its natural state as possible, there wouldn't be any need for emulsifiers, stabilizers, flavours, colours, or preservatives. And yet a great many foods that are promoted as useful in the war against weight are heavily laced with just such an array of artificial chemicals. Currently, there are only very basic rules in place regarding the amount of information a manufacturer has to declare on the packaging, so that understanding loopy labelling can be a full-time occupation, especially for anyone suffering from food intolerance or allergy or who is concerned about good health in general. In fact, it's difficult to believe that the producers don't set out deliberately to confuse. It may be true that we need to rely on at least some packaged food to feed an ever-increasing population. But do we really need the newest non-fat-fruit-flavoured-cook-in-the-pot-just-add-boiling-water-salt-free-crisps or the latest long-life-laboratory-tested-fat-free-tastes-just-like-a-home-cooked-meal-but-is-actually-recycled-sewage products? Is any of it likely to help anyone towards healthy weight loss or increased energy levels?

The only way to eat healthily and bring flavour – and, perhaps, a modicum of common sense – back into food manufacturing is to boycott the crap and go for natural, unadulterated, wholesome ingredients. In most cases, it takes no longer to prepare a meal from fresh raw items than it does to boil a polythene cod steak or heat a cardboard ready-meal. The extra time required for a few of the recipes in this book is more than made up for by the fabulous flavour and the knowledge that the food you serve is rich in real nourishment. For example, luscious pasta, flavourful fresh fish, or sumptuous stir-fries take about the same amount of time to prepare as it does to fight your way through the shrink-wrap on an E Number Pie, decide whether you should heat it with or without the cover, read every scrap of small print searching for the bit that tells you how long to cook it, wait for the oven to reach the right temperature, and then spend the rest of the evening picking out the melted plastic because you just discovered that – whoops! – the lid should be left on only if it's shrivelled in the microwave!

Weigh too high

Everyone knows that dietary guidelines and nutritional research take a 180 degree turn every other day or so, and no one can blame the consumer for being confused. In the same way that the cholesterol goal-posts have been moved so that readings once considered OK are now dangerous enough to worry you to death, every new issue of the official government height/weight chart can leave you thinking you're heavier than ever before, even if you haven't gained a single pound!

But, whatever the experts decide is right today and wrong tomorrow, one thing stands like stone. Natural, unprocessed, unadulterated fat, whether saturated or unsaturated, is not bad food, nor does it cause obesity or heart disease when taken as part of a varied, moderate diet. Unfortunately, no one seems to have noticed this. Instead, we are set on serving up any kind of synthetic, artificial, fat-reduced, fat-free, plastic-tasting, packaged garbage just so that we can look better on the beach.

The All Day Energy Diet stands for healthy eating, real food, and realistic goals. It will help you to achieve your best weight through simple lifestyle and dietary changes, by improving the digestion, enhancing energy levels, and satisfying the appetite so that cravings cease to be a problem. Nothing fancy. No impossible promises. No magic bullets. No excesses or extremes but lots of lovely grub and more than a dash of delicious indulgence. Plus plenty of tried and tested tips and hints to help you on your way.

TWO

Top tips for successful dieting

∾

1   For the time being, forget about **weighing yourself**.
    Body weight can vary by as much as six pounds between
    morning and evening whether you have eaten or
    exercised or not. If you can't live without doing so,
    weigh yourself once – on reliable scales – before you read
    the rest of this book and then don't bother again for
    several weeks. You'll soon know which way your weight
    is going by the notches in your belt or the space inside
    your waistband! The All Day Energy Diet encourages
    slow and gentle weight loss; weighing yourself too often
    will only give you a false impression of progress.

2   Make a **shopping list** before you go for the groceries. It
    helps to keep bills down and avoids the trap of buying
    not-so-healthy items. And shop after you have eaten,
    not when you're hungry. This way, you are more likely
    to buy only what you need.

3   If you are used to buying meals in packets, look to see if
    the **fresh** equivalent is available first. It will almost
    certainly be more nourishing, quicker to prepare, and
    probably cheaper!

4   Ignore foods that proclaim 'low in **cholesterol**'. It's
    nothing more than marketing hype and often an excuse
    to raise the price. The cholesterol in food does not affect
    significantly the cholesterol in blood, nor should it
    affect your weight.

5   Avoid processed, packaged **reduced-fat** foods. If you
    need yoghurt, cream, or cheese, go for the full-fat
    versions and eat half the quantity that you would
    normally eat. Low-fat equivalents are often loaded with
    artificial additives which, some experts believe, can
    cause weight increase by encouraging toxicity. Whether
    you agree or not, who needs to eat laboratory-formulated
    chemicals that have been around for such a short amount
    of time that no one knows the long-term effects?

6   Cut back on **sugar** and sugary foods but don't
    substitute artificial sweeteners. They may be calorie-free
    but researchers have now found that chemical
    sweeteners can act as appetite stimulants, making you
    want to eat more instead of less. There is also mounting
    evidence that sweeteners can cause allergic reactions in
    some people. If you drink Coke, go for occasional
    'originals' and pass on the cans of low cal. Unless you
    are diabetic, small quantities of real sugar are a better
    bet than sweeteners. Page 108 has more information on
    how to stay sweet without sugar.

7   Weight problems are often linked to a condition known
    as **candidiasis**, a condition caused by overgrowth of the
    yeast fungus *Candida albicans*. Where weight problems
    are accompanied by digestive discomfort, bloating,
    irritable bowel, hormonal disorders, skin problems,
    lethargy, poor concentration, anxiety attacks, skin
    eruptions, recurring cystitis, or headaches or migraine,
    candidiasis should be suspected. The best course of
    action under these circumstances is to consult a
    qualified nutrition practitioner who is familiar with the
    condition and its treatment. For further information –
    and how to find a practitioner – read *The Practical Guide
    to Candida* by Jane McWhirter (from the All Hallows

Foundation) and *Beat Candida* by Gill Jacobs
(Vermilion). Further details in Chapter 14.

8 Be sensible about **salt**. Salt has a nasty habit of hanging
on to water and may aggravate weight problems even if
the diet is otherwise perfect. If you suffer from
hypertension (high blood pressure) or osteoporosis
(brittle bone disease), oedema (fluid retention), or have
problems with weight gain, it's wise to avoid adding
salt to food and to watch food labels for hidden salt. It's
easy for any diet to become loaded with hidden salt; it
turns up in all kinds of packaged foods (both sweet and
savoury) including breakfast cereals, biscuits, soups,
bread, cake mixes, and stock cubes. Almost everything
that comes in cans has added salt. However, don't deny
yourself the pleasure of a salty taste on some 'essential'
treats, such as occasional crisps or chips. And do
sprinkle salt on to cooked foods such as potatoes or
cabbage if you really can't face them without. Like fat,
salt isn't bad for you if used sensibly and in
moderation.

9 Add other **flavours** to food by experimenting with
flavourful ingredients such as culinary herbs, balsamic
vinegar, sun-dried tomatoes, garlic, or ginger.

10 Be sensible about **saturates**. Despite apparently
irrefutable evidence, the jury is still out on whether
saturated fat actually does cause heart disease. Until we
know the real truth, the best advice is to avoid excesses
and extremes (either high or low) and keep fat intake at
a reasonable level. Don't deep fry anything, avoid pre-
packaged foods that are high in fat (it's probably
hydrogenated anyway), and treat take-aways as treats,
not as everyday standbys.

11 Give up **margarine** spreads that are made using the

hydrogenation process (check the label) and use either small amounts of butter or a *non*-hydrogenated margarine (available from health-food stores) for spreading. Avoid all regular cooking oils, including sunflower oil, corn oil, vegetable oil, etc. Many of them are extracted using chemical solvents (see page 25) and are considered by a number of leading health experts not to be stable enough for heating to high temperatures. For cooking, choose *extra virgin* olive oil. It costs more but is better for you and you'll need far less. Bottles labelled *pure* olive oil, by the way, will not be the best quality.

12 Achieve your low-fat diet in a **natural and healthy** way by going for lots of wholegrains, fresh fish, free-range poultry (without skin), soya, pulses, nuts, seeds, fresh vegetables and salads, organic jacket potatoes, fresh and dried fruit, free-range eggs, real cheeses, and live yoghurt made from sheep's or goat's milk.

13 **Cow's milk** may be a factor to consider if you are having problems losing weight. A common allergen and the cause of digestive discomfort in some people, it is best kept to small amounts during any weight-loss programme. Use it in tea and coffee if you don't like them black but don't drink the stuff by the glass and don't swamp your cereal in it. Soya milk makes a useful alternative but, again, can be difficult for sensitive systems to digest. Or you could make your own almond milk. Delicious on cereals and very nutritious. The method is on page 137. Even if you don't drink milk, it's unlikely that you'll lose out on calcium since so many foods are rich in this mineral. Chapter 6 has a list of the best sources.

14 If energy and staying power are a problem for you, try

giving up the breakfast toast and changing your **wheat** cereal to oats – or try gluten-free muesli. And ditch the squashy lunchtime sandwich, too. The mass-produced type of wheat used in bread and in most cereals can leave you feeling lethargic and, in some people, has been found to be the **sole cause of their weight problem**. Tuck into the delicious breakfast menu in Chapter 9.

15 Instead of the aforesaid sandwich bread, change to yeast-free soda bread, pumpernickel, or brown pitta **bread**. Some bakeries have speciality breads made with organic flour. You'll need to experiment to find out which type suits you best. Reports from patients suggest that digestion is improved and energy lifted when ordinary bread is avoided. If all bread is a problem, then go for rye crackers, rice cakes, or oat biscuits. Many crispbreads are wheat-based or have added wheat bran, so it's worth reading labels carefully.

The wheat in pasta, durum semolina, does not appear to cause the severity of digestive discomfort as bread and cereal wheat. However, if pasta is a problem for you, try substituting either kamut or spelt (old, unadulterated wheat grains) or go for rice or legume pasta – quick to cook and good for you. Find these products in specialist health-food stores or good delicatessens.

---

16 Drink plenty of **water** between meals and another glass ten minutes before each meal. It's a common misconception that drinking water will increase weight or aggravate any problems with fluid retention. In fact, taking more fresh fluids can help to reduce bloating and swelling.

17 Eat plenty of fresh **fruit** as between-meal snacks. This improves vitamin and mineral intake and helps reduce cravings. Great for preventing those mid-morning binges and mid-afternoon slumps in energy, too.

18 Don't bother with specialist diet foods, 'milk shakes', or diet drinks. They are often expensive, usually loaded with additives, hardly ever effective in the long term, and never nourishing enough substitutes for proper meals.

19 Try to **eat regularly** and, however busy you are, avoid the temptation to go all day without food. Research has confirmed that it's far easier to maintain stable weight if food intake is sensibly spaced – 'little and often' with three smaller sized main meals and two decent snacks per day.

20 Most important of all, start the day with a decent meal. **Breakfasting** like a king has a lot going for it. Your appetite is satisfied, you're unlikely to feel hungry again for several hours, you won't need cake at coffee time, and you'll have more chance of burning off the breakfast calories throughout the day. Although missing meals may seem like a great way to drop a few pounds, the opposite is true. For example, those who skip breakfast are likely to have greater difficulty losing weight than those who start the day with a decent amount of food. Breakfast eaters tend to have better health profiles, lower cholesterol levels, and less risk of cardiovascular disease. They also display improved concentration and endurance and are less inclined to make errors of judgement over normal daily tasks.

21 Large **dinners** tend to sit on your stomach and turn furtively to fat overnight. Make lunch a medium affair and supper a light one.

22 There is good news and bad news about **chocolate**. The really bad news? The 1995 report from the Working Party on Pesticide Residues found that 82 per cent of UK-made non-organic chocolate contained residues of the pesticide Lindane (now banned in several countries but still allowed in the UK). And, according to information provided by the Women's Environmental Network, the cocoa crop is one of the most heavily contaminated with pesticides and other artificial chemicals.

If you love the stuff, choose the new organic varieties made by Green & Black. They are absolutely delicious and available from most supermarkets, health-food stores and delicatessens. Treat yourself to a square or two after the main meal of the day. You'll enjoy it thoroughly but are less likely to pig out on a whole bar if you have just eaten a substantial meal. And if you're worried about the caffeine content, don't be. Compared to the 150mg in an average cup of coffee, chocolate contains only 6mg per ounce. (Chapter 12.)

It flatters you for a while; it warms you for an instant; then suddenly it kindles a mortal fever in you.

> The Marquise de Sévigné on chocolate

Another 'plus' for chocolate is that it never seems to cause spotty skin in doctors or dermatologists (they don't think it's a problem). However, acne sufferers say different. Sorry to be a misery but if you are prone to break-outs, all kinds of chocolate are best avoided.

23 Eat more '**brown**' foods. Swap white rice for brown rice. Up your intake of brown pasta. Go for yeast-free wholemeal soda bread, rye bread, pumpernickel (black rye), or brown pitta bread instead of the usual squidgy loaf. Wholerye crackers, oat biscuits, and rice cakes are good (wheat-free) sources of dietary fibre too. (Sorry, but the 'brown is best' rule doesn't apply to sugar. Nutritionally, brown sugar is no better than white unless it is unrefined cane sugar or molasses.)

24 Include plenty of **dietary fibre**; it is good for helping to keep cholesterol in check, encouraging a balanced blood glucose, satisfying the appetite, and maintaining a merry morning smile. Steer clear of wheat bran which can cause general digestive discomfort, heartburn, colic, bloating, fatigue, grouchy temper, irritable bowel syndrome, and even constipation in some people. Oats, rye, and brown rice are good sources of roughage. So are many fresh fruits and vegetables, split peas, chick peas, lentils, all kinds of beans, potato skins (organic only), brown pasta, dried fruit (especially figs), nuts, and seeds. The best regulated households also use either a daily tablespoonful of linseeds (try Linusit Gold) or psyllium husk fibre with a tumbler of water. Find these vital ingredients in your health-food store.

> Did you know ... that figs contain more dietary fibre than wheat bran or earth-moving prunes? Fresh or dried, figs are rich in calcium and potassium. Dried figs make a terrific sweet treat and are good to carry with you in case of uncontrollable hunger.

25 Take mealtimes seriously. Make **time** to feed. If you find this a difficult new habit to get into because of your schedule, keep a diary of your activities for seven

days and, at the end of the week, sit down and decide which of the tasks that took you away from proper eating could be restructured (or given up). You owe it to your long-term health and well-being to look after yourself. Don't allow your mealtimes to be disrupted by the demands of other people. If a family member at your table or someone at work needs something during your meal, why not suggest that they fetch whatever it is themselves or wait until you have finished eating?

26 If you have a tendency to 'pig out', try this trick. Measure your dinner **plates** and then go out and buy a set of smaller ones. Meals will still seem sizeable but portions are slightly smaller.

27 Avoid **colours** that are known to stimulate the appetite. Don't use red, orange, or yellow plates, tableware, napkins, or cutlery. If your dining area is painted in any of these colours, change it. Go for green, turquoise, or light blue.

28 Look upon any foods made with **white flour** or **white sugar** as occasional treats. New research shows that foods such as white bread, pastries, cakes and sweet treats are linked to a condition known as insulin resistance (a precursor to diabetes) and to obesity. It has been estimated by some researchers that insulin resistance affects 25 per cent of the (non-diabetic) population. (See Chapter 4 for more info on blood sugar problems.) In addition, research now suggests that fats and sugars eaten together may be far more of a health hazard than fat alone and that cutting out fat won't help long-term weight loss if these refined starches still figure prominently in the diet.

29 Forget calorie counting and portion weighing. Just let your **natural appetite** tell you when you are

comfortably full. If you find this a problem, The All Day Energy Diet recipes should help satisfy your hunger.

30 Improve your **digestion**. Many weight problems are made worse because food is poorly digested and inadequately absorbed. Sit down to meals and rest for ten minutes after the last mouthful. Eating slowly and chewing each mouthful thoroughly help to satisfy your appetite without needing to overeat. If your weight problem is accompanied by digestive discomfort, hiatus hernia, heartburn, or any kind of bowel disorder, give serious thought to food combining as a way of improving health and reducing weight. *The Food Combining Diet* or *Food Combining in 30 Days* are very easy to follow, step-by-step guides (see Chapter 14).

31 Don't overdo the **alcohol** but don't abstain unnecessarily. Beer and spirits are best avoided but a glass of dry wine with a main meal is positively encouraged. According to a report in the *American Journal of Clinical Nutrition*, food consumed with alcoholic beverages may be more fattening than those without. Apparently, we also spend more time at the table if we drink than if we don't. But wine (especially red) can help the digestion and may be good for the heart too; so don't be too quick to jump on the wagon. Just be sensible about intake.

32 Take more **exercise** but don't go to silly extremes. Exhausting your already exhausted body by working out for more than an hour a day is unlikely to help you to lose any more weight than if you pace yourself sensibly. If you're not into strenuous exercise, be comforted by the fact that a twenty- to thirty-minute brisk walk each day (or forty to sixty minutes three times a week) is a perfectly adequate way to begin your new

programme. Diet and exercise go together. It really is true that physical activity fosters a healthy body. Eat healthily, too, and you'll feel more like indulging in physical activity.

33 If you are tied to the home or your timetable really doesn't allow you to get outside to exercise, consider the possibility of **home exercise equipment**. Could you find space in the spare room, garage, or shed for a treadmill, rowing machine, rebounder (mini-trampoline), or stationary bike? According to a study carried out in the Sports Performance Laboratory at Wisconsin Medical College, treadmill activity burned off more calories (700 per hour) than other equipment, possibly because it involved more natural body movement. But, the researchers point out, all the machines were good at helping weight loss and improving fitness levels. Over the long term, they advise, it's what the person exercising enjoys most, finds most comfortable, and is willing to stick to that is best for their health.

34 If your exercise routine is more strenuous (i.e. long runs, extended sessions at the gym) but you are finding that you have a tendency to run out of **oomph** more quickly than perhaps you should, some minor adjustments to the diet can help. Surprisingly, although we read a lot about the benefits of complex carbohydrates, starchy foods aren't always the best choice to sustain energy levels. Some starches, such as bread wheat – and the modified starch that is added to many processed foods – are not well digested and can contribute to abdominal bloating and discomfort.

35 Check that your diet isn't too low in **fat**. This may sound strange advice when we are almost overwhelmed with advice on how to cut fat intake. New thinking in sports nutrition suggests that adding a bit more fat to some meals may help endurance and performance. Include carbohydrates such as pasta, jacket potatoes, oats, and brown rice; avoid processed fats but add little extras such as small amounts of butter, olive oil, cheeses, and full-fat yoghurt to your diet, especially on exercise days. Steer clear of low-fat products that contain modified starch, i.e. as in some reduced-fat foods. It's added to give bulk and some of the structure which was lost when the fat was removed, but has been referred to as being 'no better nutritionally than wallpaper paste'.

36 Start a basic **supplement** programme when you start The All Day Energy Diet. Recommendations are in Chapter 6.

37 Don't be shy about seeing your **doctor** for a check-up. If you've been fighting the flab for years without success, have symptoms of lethargy, persistent tiredness, depression, constipation, hair loss, reduced or non-existent sex drive, high cholesterol, high blood pressure, or dry skin, ask for a full blood profile and a test for thyroid function, and women should ask for the test to include all female hormones. An underactive thyroid gland can cause weight problems but often goes undetected because it isn't picked up in standard tests. Ask for TSH (thyroid stimulating hormone) to be tested for as well. Many doctors still only check the levels of thyroid hormone circulating in the blood, a measurement that doesn't always detect early hypothyroidism, the medical term for underactive thyroid. The condition contributes to obesity by slowing the metabolic rate so that fewer and fewer

calories are burned off, irrespective of how much you eat or how much you exercise. If you are not satisfied with the results, ask about the Basal Temperature Test (BTT) pioneered in the United States by Dr Broda Barnes and listed in the United States doctors' 'bible', *The Physician's Desk Reference*. A simple procedure that can be carried out at home, the BTT is based on the fact that body temperature in those with thyroid malfunction can be persistently lower than average. By collecting temperatures over several days, a trained eye can determine whether a thyroid problem exists and take action to treat accordingly.

38 Don't be persuaded to take **appetite suppressants** or any kind of weight-loss drug unless you are receiving support and advice from your doctor, hospital specialist or dietician. Medication hardly ever provides the answer to healthy weight loss. Nor does it work on everyone. The latest anti-obesity drug to be launched in the USA is supposed to suppress appetite by reducing serotonin levels in the brain. Even though a major study of 900 overweight people demonstrated only minimal weight loss, the promoters see it as 'an important milestone in the war on fat'. Obesity experts are more cautious and say that weight management drugs will never be able to turn a size 18 into a size 8. Nor will they work without significant commitment to lifestyle changes that include diet modification and exercise.

39 If all else fails and you are not making any progress, consider an appointment with a qualified **nutritionist** who can test for allergies. It is common for food intolerance to trigger weight problems. A good nutrition practitioner should also be familiar with Dr Barnes' Basal Temperature Test. See Chapter 12 for details of how to find a qualified therapist.

40 If you are a **smoker** but reluctant to give up because
you think you'll put weight on, The All Day Energy
Diet should help you to quit the weed and stay trim.
There is good evidence that increasing the intake of
alkaline-forming foods (i.e. fresh fruits, salads,
vegetables, and juices) can reduce the craving for
nicotine. Anything that leads to an increase in the
body's acid balance (stress is an example) increases the
craving, too. Taking on board more fresh produce ups
the alkaline balance and consequently seems to reduce
the hankering for cigarettes. Nearly all fruits and
vegetables are helpful; particularly good are beetroot,
beet greens, carrots, celery, broccoli, cauliflower,
cauliflower greens, onions, fresh herbs, potatoes, sweet
potatoes, spinach, watercress, apples, kiwi fruit, grapes,
grapefruit, and cherries.

In addition, the average weight increase experienced
by quitting smokers is only ten pounds – certainly not
enough to make a thin person fat or to increase the risk
of coronary heart disease. Smoking is far more of a risk
to life than a bit of extra padding. Health experts
estimate that you'd have to put on ten times that
amount (nearly seven stone) to be at the same danger
level as you were when you were smoking. But I'm not
here to nag you about it. You already know the
dangers; that cigarettes cause premature ageing, use up
enormous amounts of vitamins and minerals, contain
huge numbers of cancer-causing chemicals initiating
extensive free radical damage, cause more than two
million deaths per year in so-called advanced Western
society alone, and, most worrying of all, trigger serious
health problems in non-smokers too.

Here's what to do if you're really keen to stop smoking:

- Start The All Day Energy Diet and follow it for four weeks BEFORE you pick a quit day for your cigarettes. Write the chosen date in your diary and, once decided upon, stick to it. Continue to follow the diet (and the supplement programme recommended in Chapter 6) once you've given up smoking.
- Cut down on alcohol while you're trying to quit. Booze increases the body's acidity and so makes it more difficult to manage without nicotine. Steer clear of spirits, beer, and fortified wine.
- Up your daily activity level. Go for a brisk walk each morning or evening. Walk fast for thirty minutes a day.
- Let the lift go without you and take the stairs. Or walk up the escalator instead of letting it walk you.
- Get into the breakfast habit. Many smokers skip breakfast in favour of the first cigarette. Chewing food gives the mouth something to do!
- Invest in a juicing machine and start your day with freshly made juice. Try kiwi and grape, apple and celery, mango and papaya, or any fruit combination that you enjoy. Drink the juice first thing before bathing and then eat breakfast once you're dressed. In the evening, make vegetable or fruit juice mixes while you are waiting for the main meal. Prepare a particularly healthy alkalizing combination with one apple, one fresh raw beetroot (not the precooked, preserved kind), two carrots (organic only), and a handful of seedless grapes (black or green). (It is truly delicious. If you include beetroot, don't forget to wear an apron!)
- Make sure your diet includes plenty of fresh fruits and vegetables that are rich in protective antioxidants.
- Eat fresh fruit between meals, i.e. mid-morning and mid-

afternoon. Apples and grapes are good. Or chomp on raw carrots or nibble at unblanched almonds and dried figs. They all help to reduce cravings.

- If you're desperate, chew gum. But go for the original stuff and avoid brands that contain artificial sweetening.
- Keep your hands busy. Take up a hobby such as pottery, painting, or gardening.
- Although most smokers look forward to a cigarette after meals, the craving for nicotine can be worse when you are hungry, tired, or stressed. Eating regular meals and going to bed at a sensible hour may seem like very basic advice but it's worth reiterating if you are fighting to give up smoking.
- After meals (a particularly favourite time for smoking), use the time to floss your teeth or use toothpicks.
- Keep a drink of water or juice alongside you, or, if you're travelling, carry a small flask or bottle. Sip at it every time you fancy a smoke.
- Don't dismiss the possibility of nicotine gum or patches to get you over the hump. They are not a terrific solution in the long term but can help you through the darkest days.
- Follow the supplement recommendations in Chapter 6 or, at the very least, take a good quality multivitamin/mineral or antioxidant supplement together with an additional 2g of vitamin C complex every day. Your health-food store should have an extensive range of products, or you can order by mail or phone from the list in Chapter 12.
- Research shows that fish oils may be particularly helpful to smokers. If you are not eating fresh oily fish twice a week, add fish oil capsules to your supplement programme. If you are unable to take fish or fish oil for any reason, include linseeds or linseed oil capsules. Chapter 12 has more information.

41 Above all, *walk* your weight-loss programme in small
steps. In other words, *don't rush at it*. **Take your time**.
Introduce one or two changes per day or per week,
depending upon how much time you have available.
Before you begin, spend an hour or two just strolling
around your supermarket, delicatessen, grocery store,
and health-food shop familiarizing yourself with their
stock. Use this knowledge to increase the variety in
your diet. Don't be afraid to ask for advice on foods that
you'd like to try but that are unfamiliar. For new ideas
on what to look out for and what's best avoided, read
Chapter 7 on Getting Started.

42 Once you've begun your new eating plan, **aim** to lose
around two pounds each week or half a stone a month.
Shed the weight more quickly than that and it's far less
likely to stay off! Remember that The All Day Energy
Diet works best if used in conjunction with a sensible
exercise programme.

Before you begin any exercise programme, diet plan or supplement
package, see your GP for a check-up.

Part Two

Superhealth Benefits of The All Day Energy Diet

THREE

Boosting brainpower

❧

IMPROVE CONCENTRATION
RELIEVE DEPRESSION
LIFT MOOD
VITAL VITAMINS AND MINERALS
HOW EXERCISE HELPS THE BRAIN TO FUNCTION
HOW TO STAY SHARP AND SLEEP WELL

❧

Brain, *n.* An apparatus with which we think we think.
Ambrose Bierce (1842–1914), American writer and
journalist, in *The Devil's Dictionary*

Food affects not only the way we feel but how efficiently we function. It can determine whether we are happy, ratty, or depressed and will also influence attitude, alertness, concentration and memory. It's well known that someone who is wide awake will store and consolidate short- and long-term memories far more efficiently than anyone mentally exhausted. When an energy crisis strikes, one of the first faculties to fail is information storage and recall. If we are under pressure, working long hours, not getting proper rest, rarely able to relax, and not eating as well as we could, brain cells become addled and exhausted too.

I'm sure you know the feeling well.

- Vital bits of information that are stowed away safely in the memory bank just *won't* come to the surface.
- When concentration and co-ordination suffer, the mind wanders.
- You put things down and then, ten minutes later, can't find them. You lose important personal effects like keys and credit cards and only call off an Interpol investigation when they turn up right where you know you'd already searched several times!
- Appointments appear in your diary on completely the wrong day and you don't even recall writing anything down. You can't remember what you just read. (Ah ha! Proves you need this book!)
- Normal everyday items begin to attack you: you bump into door handles, try to push instead of pull, head for the opening that says 'Exit Only', take the up escalator and then can't find one that goes down.
- You meet someone in the high street who you know extremely well but simply can't put a name to the face.
- You go shopping and come home with only half the things you went for.

I've met many people who worry that this loss of mental agility may be the first signs of their trolley coming off the track. A much more likely explanation is that their brain cells are overworked to the point of complete exhaustion.

We can only access stored data from our brain if signals are sent and received correctly. For this to happen, brain cells need feeding. Neurotransmitters, chemical messengers that fire information from the brain throughout the nervous system require a constant supply of certain nutrients in order to function efficiently. The brain also has complete priority over the rest of the body when it comes to nourishment. In other words, the nutrients you take on board will be used first for brain business and only then for other body functions.

The thinking person's workout

Did you know that, although the average brain weighs only 2–3 per cent of total bodyweight, it needs around half of the oxygen inhaled to function efficiently. The more aerobic exercise you take and the more efficiently you breathe, the better the circulation of blood and nutrients to the brain.

Exercise doesn't just help us physically. It also improves mood and attitude, reduces anxiety, depression and tension, helps overcome phobias, and increases motivation. It can enhance energy levels and improve general health, too.

A link is well established between physical activity and a reduced risk of cardiovascular disease. Exercise helps to keep arteries and veins free of gunge and so contributes to improved circulation and blood flow to the brain. No wonder there is also a link between absence of heart disease and an active mind.

Other observed benefits are better emotional stability, increased assertiveness, improved coping skills, and greater sexual satisfaction!

The speed of someone's reactions declines with age. So too does the ability to process information. However, researchers have found that being involved in regular physical activity (brisk walking or swimming, for example) slows down age-related mental decline. In addition to the actual exercise, getting out and about, seeing people, holding conversation, and observing and acknowledging what goes on around us all help to keep the brain supplied with information. The old adage 'Use it or lose it' may, it seems, also apply to thinking!

In a study of university professors carried out in the United States, those who took regular physical exercise were able to process information faster and more efficiently than colleagues who were sedentary.

It's never too late to start exercising. Even if you've been a slob all your life, you can still reap the benefits of improved mental functioning by beginning a regular exercise programme now. However, if you haven't exercised regularly for years – or ever – first see your GP and then a qualified exercise instructor for a fitness check before you begin!

If you are unable to exercise because you're housebound, wheelchair bound or in some other way limited by disability, don't despair. Simple breathing and stretching exercises are also extremely beneficial to brain function. Your GP may be able to assist by putting you in touch with the physiotherapy department of your local hospital who can then advise on a suitable exercise programme.

Read, mark, learn, and inwardly digest

What you eat – and how well you digest it – can have a profound effect on mental acuity and agility. Eat the right foods in the right combinations and it is perfectly possible to pep up your brainpower and enhance performance. Research suggests that foods can produce beneficial effects by interacting with the body's natural daily rhythms of waking, working, and winding down. It's long been theorized that starchy foods are sedative. If you've had the worst of days and need something to relax you before sleep, scientists now suggest that a meal based on complex carbohydrates such as potatoes, pasta, or rice may be more soporific than a large Scotch! Calming carbs are not such a great idea, however, if you've planned a night of unrivalled passion and would prefer to be up and at it. (See Chapter 5 if you'd rather be gymnastic than somnambulistic!)

Sweet dreams?

Even that highly refined carbohydrate, sugar – which we have so long believed to be an instant energy booster – has been found in studies to bring on fatigue and drowsiness. The sugar fix may appear to give us energy by quickly raising the levels of glucose in the blood and satiating hunger. Like any stimulant, however, the effect is short-lived and can leave us feeling even more drained and lethargic than before. However, the *comfort* to be had from eating something sweet shouldn't be denied and does have basis in scientific fact. Although the old wives and grannies who recommended a spoonful of honey to induce sleep didn't know why it worked, it's now known that foods rich in sugar speed up production of a calming brain chemical called serotonin, the effects of which can be felt in as little time as half an hour.

Pass your exam on protein

Proteins, on the other hand, have been linked to motivation and clear thinking and are the best foods to choose if you want to stay sharp and observant. Take two groups of people and feed one lot the starchy stuff and the others a meal of turkey, chicken, eggs, or cheese and, researchers tell us, you'll usually find those on the proteins to be far more alert and awake. This doesn't mean that sleepy people should avoid starch or that those with plenty of pep should stay permanently on protein. Far from it. A balanced diet is absolutely crucial to balanced health and that means including as wide a variety of foods as possible.

But mixing – or not mixing – certain foods at certain mealtimes can make a real difference to your day – and night. Instead of lying awake, you could be sleeping like a log. And rather than crashing out like a comatose couch potato by lunchtime, you could be feeling full of energy. Understanding the way in which certain foods affect you as an individual is a simple way to modify mood and enhance general well-being.

Vitamins and minerals for memory

Whether or not additional nutrients can improve learning ability remains a controversial area. Although it's unlikely that taking tons of vitamin pills will result in immediate membership of Mensa, it seems likely that, where deficiencies occur, the regular use of quality nutrient supplements improves concentration and, possibly, recall, especially where the diet is in some way inadequate, i.e. if calories are restricted or meals missed. Chapter 6 has details.

Improving concentration and recall

Upgrading the diet, removing a few problem foods, and adding some extra healthy ones can go a long way to enhancing attention span and co-ordination.

One supplement that has proved to be extremely helpful in this area is **Ginkgo biloba**. Studies have shown ginkgo to be able to improve blood flow to the brain, as well as enhancing the general circulation, alleviating the problem of cold hands and feet. I have found ginkgo (together with evening primrose oil or borage oil GLA supplements) to be an excellent treatment for Raynaud's phenomena (narrowed arteries in fingers and toes in response to cold).

Improved blood supply to the brain provides brain cells with more oxygen and glucose (brain fuel), counteracting symptoms such as poor concentration, poor recall, and loss of memory, while, at the same time, lifting lethargy. In addition, the active ingredients in ginkgo reduce the risk of blood clots, support the nervous system and provide antioxidant protection to brain cells. Ginkgo biloba is available in tablet and capsule form. Chapter 12 has details of suppliers.

Foods to fight depression

Feeling down in the dumps every now and then is perfectly normal. It happens to us all and is a natural balance to better days. But if depression, dolefulness, or gloom and doom are commonplace, it could be worth examining the diet in a bit more detail. Various population studies suggest that borderline deficiencies of certain vitamins and minerals are common. People aren't so lacking in nourishment that they are falling apart at the seams from obvious malnutrition but, nevertheless, may be suffering from subclinical levels of a wide range of nutrients. Symptoms may be numerous and varied but inconsistent and not considered serious enough to warrant further investigation.

Vital vitamins

A good example of a vitamin vital to brain function is the B vitamin folic acid. Not getting enough of this can lead to insomnia, poor memory, fatigue, and irritability. A deficiency of vitamin B1 (thiamin) is known to bring on similar symptoms of fatigue and bad-temper. Low levels of riboflavin (vitamin B2) can mean poor memory. Where vitamin B6 is lacking, there may be higher levels of a chemical called homocysteine, now regarded as a risk factor for heart disease. Elevated homocysteine is also associated with impaired memory function and poor co-ordination, and a link has been established between depression and cardiovascular disease. In another set of tests, subjects who had the lowest levels of B12 and folic acid were unable to memorize or copy the simplest drawings of rectangles or cubes.

Making sure that the diet contains foods rich in B group vitamins and supplementing with B complex capsules or tablets should not be looked upon as a cure-all or magic bullet but has led to speedy improvements in a number of cases. One group of women suffering with mood swings and irritability were supplemented with B group vitamins and reported feeling better within a month.

Where to find the best sources of B group vitamins

Apricots	Good multivitamin
Avocado pear	supplements
B complex supplements	Green leafy vegetables
Bananas	Lamb's kidney
Brown rice	Lamb's liver
Carrots	Legumes
Cheese	Milk
Dried fruits	Nuts
Free-range chicken	Oats
Free-range eggs	Oily fish

Pumpkin
Root vegetables (carrots and
  potatoes are good sources
  of Bs)

Rye flour
Soy flour
Spirulina
Yoghurt

Did you know that ... vitamin B1 is the most unstable member of the B group, easily lost when frozen food is thawed or the nutrient is leached into cooking water.

Understanding 'E' numbers

Not all E numbers are bad news. For example, riboflavin (vitamin B2), the ingredient in multivitamin products that turns urine (harmlessly) orange, deep yellow or orangey-green, is also used to produce natural orange/yellow colour to food. You'll see it on some food labels as **E101**. Take care not to confuse it with the less than desirable **E110** Sunset Yellow colour, a common ingredient in many packaged foods that is made from synthetic coal-tar dye and can cause skin rashes, gastric upset, and sickness. To avoid confusion, it can be useful to invest in a pocket guide to E numbers and carry it with you when shopping (see Chapter 14).

Vital minerals

Studies show that the trace mineral **selenium** improves mood and helps to lift depression and anxiety. Symptoms are more pronounced in countries where soil selenium is low. Levels in food depend to a large extent on how much selenium occurs naturally in the soil. Food processing also destroys selenium. For example, brown rice may have up to fifteen times more of this mineral than white rice.

	Where to find selenium	
Antioxidant supplements	Fresh vegetables	Seafood
Chicken liver	Lamb's kidney	Sunflower seeds
Fish	Lamb's liver	Sweetbreads
Free-range eggs	Lean meat	Wholegrains
Fresh fruits	Multimineral supplements	

Zinc is another trace element needed for cognitive function; in other words, being aware, recognizing, noticing. Find this mineral in seafood, fish, pulses, wholegrains, lamb's liver, oysters, cheese, eggs, rice, potatoes, green beans, and tomatoes. A 'worth taking' multimineral or antioxidant supplement label should declare around 50mg to 100mg of zinc by weight or 7mg to 15mg of *elemental* (usable) zinc.

Boron is yet another important trace element which has received recent publicity due to its possible role in the treatment of arthritis and osteoporosis. But boron is also involved in the brain's electrical activity. It's needed only in tiny amounts but deficiencies can lead to sluggishness, poor recognition, and reduced mental alertness. Good natural sources are green vegetables, fresh fruit, nuts, and pulses. Boron also turns up in good quality mineral products.

Calcium, magnesium, and **potassium** are important to the brain, being involved in the transmission of nerve impulses.

Where to find calcium

Brown rice	Nuts	Sunflower seeds
Canned fish	Oats	Tahini
Cheese	Pulses	Tofu
Dried fruits	Stock made from	Yoghurt
Most vegetables	bones	

Where to find magnesium

Brown and white	as apples,	Nuts
pasta	bananas, and	Pulses
Brown rice	grapefruit	Seafood
Dried fruits	Fresh ginger	Wholegrains
Fish	Green vegetables	
Fresh fruit such	Lemon juice	

Where to find potassium

Blackstrap	Fresh ginger	beverages, e.g.
molasses	Fresh vegetables and	Bioforce,
Dried fruits	salads	Bambu
Fresh fruits and	Garlic	Soya flour
juices	Grain-based	Wholegrains

Chapter 6 has information on how to choose the best supplements for fighting fatigue, lifting energy, and improving mood.

Cholesterol – can levels be too low?

Fat has long been associated with obesity, heart disease, and elevated cholesterol. Unfortunately, although many of us still eat far too much fat, others have taken the 'fat is bad' message to unhealthy extremes. The right kind of low-fat diet is probably a very good idea but one made up of processed, packaged low-fat foods may not be. A 'no fat' diet is likely to be extremely unhealthy, especially in the long term. Current wisdom has it that saturated fat raises cholesterol but there is far more to eating healthily than avoiding butter and lard. For one thing, experts now believe that striving for a low cholesterol level could be counter-productive. If you've been trying hard to reduce yours, don't lower it too far. Apart from the fact that perfect readings don't always equate with less risk of heart disease, there is good evidence to show that when levels fall too low (either through diet or medication) there is a greater likelihood of depression, black moods, and premature death by accident or injury – or even suicide. Tests carried out on subjects with a history of violence towards others have been found to have lower than normal levels of certain fats, including cholesterol, in the blood. In addition, cholesterol is an important nutrient in its own right, being used in the production of serotonin, the brain chemical I mentioned earlier (page 55).

Some fat in the diet is needed to provide the fatty vitamins and essential fatty acids (EFAs) that are so vital to efficient brain function and nerve transmission. Scientists are still working on finding the actual physical dysfunction that leads to depression, but do know already that it involves the neurotransmitters which carry signals across the synapse (the junction between one nerve and another) or from a nerve ending to a gland or muscle. When the fat composition of the diet is altered, the effectiveness of the transmitted information via the synapses also changes. Efficient synapses can amplify messages through nerves a thousandfold. It's clear that certain types of unsaturated fatty acids (especially those found in oily fish) can lift depression, but that where the diet is low in essential fatty acids, 'the blues' are more common.

Best sources of essential fatty acids

GLA supplements based on borage oil or evening primrose oil

Cold pressed food oils

(e.g. safflower, walnut)

Fish oil supplements

Nutritional grade linseed oil supplements

Oily fish

Quality seeds such as sunflower, pumpkin, and linseeds

Whole fresh nuts

Fixing fatigue with caffeine

When it comes to instant energy boosters, coffee is probably the best known pick-you-up. Although it's common to hear people talk in terms of caffeine causing a surge of adrenalin, latest studies suggest that coffee actually 'stimulates' by *suppressing* production of calming chemicals, leading to faster reaction times and increased concentration. People who drink a cup of coffee after lunch generally have a longer attention span than those who abstain. However, moderation is the key here. Professional coffee drinkers who take more than three cups at one sitting or sup the stuff all day seem to be less attentive and more prone to lethargy. So if you're wondering how to quantify excess, more than three cups of coffee (or tea) per day is probably too much – one cup a day is the target to aim for. Be honest about your intake. If it's too high, cut back a cup at a time over a period of several weeks so that you don't notice any withdrawal symptoms. Consider substituting other drinks such as Caro or Bambu or other grain-based coffee substitutes, more juices, and definitely more water.

Top tip for tip-top alertness

Always eat breakfast. If you have a heavy day ahead and need to be 'up together', go for something that will keep you nourished for several hours. Studies show that those who miss breakfast are more likely to lose concentration and make mistakes in normal daily tasks. They also have a tendency towards higher cholesterol levels, obesity and greater risk of heart disease and stroke than people whose morning meal is substantial. If there is a chance you might miss lunch, choose a cooked breakfast, preferably one that contains protein such as eggs or fish. Chapter 9 has some super-sustaining breakfast suggestions. Toast (even when it's whole-meal) tends to zap energy and, on its own, won't satisfy the appetite for long. If you are finding lately that, come 10.30am, you're drooling over your packed lunch or wishing yourself away to the canteen or coffee shop then it's possible that your breakfast doesn't contain enough quality calories.

FOUR

Making maximum energy

჻

HELP FOR HYPOGLYCAEMIA
UNDERSTANDING SWEET TEMPTATIONS
ENERGY SUPPLEMENTS

჻

> In 1872, an English sugar merchant named Henry Tate patented a
> method of cutting sugar into little cubes. Much of the fortune he
> made as a result was used to purchase a collection of paintings
> now housed in London's Tate Gallery.

One important key to keeping energy levels high is to ensure
that the balance of glucose in your blood remains relatively
constant. As low blood glucose has been linked so often to
energy problems (and can be a particular thorn in the side of
anyone who is trying to lose weight on a low-calorie diet), it's
worth taking a moment to understand the mechanism that
keeps this very special body fuel in check.

Energy is produced within the body from the food we eat
but, before it can be utilized, it must first be 'processed' –
just as petrol is from oil.

The main type of body fuel is glucose, not the kind you
find in sweets, drinks, or glucose tablets but a special type

that is essential for all physical activity. Glucose is converted, primarily, from carbohydrates (starchy and sugary foods) and is kept in balance by various hormones. When it enters the bloodstream following digestion, levels of blood glucose rise. This is natural and happens to everyone. In response, insulin is produced by the pancreas to return the blood glucose level (BGL) to what is considered normal balance, drawing the excess into storage.

When glucose is not needed for immediate use, it is transferred to liver and muscle tissues and stored as glycogen to ensure reserve supplies of energy for the next twelve to twenty-four hours. If there is too much glucose around and the liver and muscle cells become saturated, any overload will be converted into fat. As soon as levels fall to a point where they are about to slip below normal, other hormones are brought into play to restore the *status quo*. By this clever system, the quantity of circulating glucose is kept in check.

In certain cases, however, the balancing mechanism doesn't function as it should, leading to a condition known as *hypoglycaemia* (hypo = low, glycaemia = blood glucose). In some sensitive individuals, insulin may be secreted to excess. Where large amounts of it are floating around in the blood, the BGL falls too far, too rapidly – a condition known as *hyper-insulin-ism* (simply, 'too much insulin'). Tests can show insulin to be at normal levels but there may be evidence of cells having a reduced sensitivity to the hormone. In other words, they don't respond unless large quantities of insulin are produced. Sugar levels may then rise for long periods of time only to fall rapidly below normal. When BGL plummets, other hormones, including glucagon, also from the pancreas, and adrenalin and cortisol from the adrenal glands, are called up to bring the glucose levels to normal.

Common symptoms of hypoglycaemia and hyperinsulinism are sudden fatigue, lethargy, sweats, irritability, hunger, poor co-ordination, poor concentration, mid-morning and mid-afternoon slumps of energy, tearfulness, irrational thoughts, shakes, palpitations, depression, and cravings – often for sugary or salty foods. Unchecked or untreated hypoglycaemia/hyperinsulinism may eventually trigger diabetes.

Some experts believe hypoglycaemia to have reached epidemic proportions; others think the whole condition is exaggerated and applies only in a handful of cases. Whatever the eventual result of any further studies, it seems clear that symptoms similar to those of low blood glucose are common both in dieters and in that other desperate group, the permanently exhausted!

Clinical experience shows that treating the hypo, by improving dietary habits and adding a sensible supplement programme, can enhance and maintain energy levels, eliminate the cycle of craving and bingeing, and bring weight to within normal limits. The Top Tips for Successful Dieting (Chapter 2) are designed not only to trigger gentle weight loss in those who need to shed a few pounds but are also extremely helpful in treating the unpleasant effects of low blood sugar. The hints listed below in Sweet Temptations should also be worth putting into practice.

Important Note: Feedback from a number of non-insulin-dependent diabetic patients suggests that similar eating plans to those that appear in The All Day Energy Diet have improved control and reduced the need for medication. Diabetics are not advised, however, to follow any kind of diet without the support and advice of their GP, dietician or hospital consultant.

Sweet temptations

Understanding starches

To deal successfully with hypoglycaemia and the dreaded cravings, it's vital to understand the difference between basic food groups, especially between complex and refined carbohydrates (also known as starches). Think what happens when you ignite fuel in a wood-burning stove. 'Complex' fuel (e.g. logs) burn steadily and give off comfortable warmth ('energy') over a long period of time. Refined carbs could be likened to sheets of paper that when burned produce heat and flame very quickly but only for a short time.

Most highly processed foods, i.e. those made with white flour and/or sugar, come under the heading of refined carbohydrates – including cakes, biscuits, buns, doughnuts, sweets, white bread, low-fibre/sugar-coated breakfast cereals, ice-cream, chocolate, and glucose drinks as well as (brown or white) sprinkling sugar. Complex carbohydrates (wholegrain and fibrous foods such as unrefined oats, wholewheat pasta, pulses, potato skins, brown rice) are healthier because they pass less rapidly through the digestive system with the result that the natural sugars they contain are absorbed more slowly.

Refined carbohydrates are known to disturb blood glucose balance because the body is able to use them (like the burning paper) to produce instant energy, pushing very fast acting sugars into the bloodstream, initiating a hasty, sometimes excessive, insulin reaction. It seems like a good idea at the time, especially if you have hit a hunger patch, have the concentration of a supermarket trolley, and your co-ordination is all over the place! All these foods can bring about an almost miraculous rise in energy. Unfortunately, by causing such frequent swings, hormones are over-produced and undue strain is put upon the liver, the pancreas, and the adrenal system, leading to energy loss and exhaustion.

The stress which results from this type of overloading can deplete supplies of vitamin C, a major anti-stress nutrient. Stress also uses up B group vitamins that are essential for the metabolism of carbohydrates. Ironically, many refined foods already have these nutrients stripped from them during the manufacturer's processing.

Under the circumstances, it's easy to see that refined carbohydrates are not good news for good health. There is absolutely no need to abstain totally from those gooey, sticky pleasures like cream cakes and chocolate, but be sensible and treat them as treats, not everyday foods.

Concentrate on wholegrains (unrefined oats, oat biscuits, brown rice, buckwheat, whole rye, brown pasta, lentil or rice pasta) and other foods rich in fibre (jacket potatoes, split peas, beans, lentils, chickpeas, nuts, seeds, and vegetables). Pulses, avocados, and Jerusalem artichokes seem to be particularly useful foods when it comes to keeping blood glucose on an even keel.

Sneaky sugars

Watch out for hidden sugars. Foods labelled 'sucrose free' may still be loaded with glucose, maltose, dextrose or lactose; in fact, anything ending in 'ose' is a sugar of some kind. If you are trying to avoid sugar, be sure to check the packaging in detail.

Fruit and fruit juices contain fructose, an easily absorbable type of sugar. Some authorities recommend that hypo-glycaemics should eat fruit only with other foods so that

> Sugar has received a bad press as the cause of dental caries. But fruit (although good for you) can be a worse culprit. Don't stop eating fruit – the answer is to slosh water around your mouth and through your teeth after eating it to wash away the fruit sugar and acid. The same tip applies to any fresh fruit juices, fruit-flavoured drinks or cans of fizz.

the fruit sugar is absorbed more slowly. Unfortunately, this habit (although, of course, not seriously harmful) can cause digestive discomfort. It may also reduce the number of nutri-ents absorbed.

The good news is that fructose does not put anything like the same strain on the body's hormones as do other sugars (i.e. sucrose) because it doesn't need to trigger insulin pro-duction before it can be transported to the liver. In addition, most fresh fruit contains a certain amount of dietary fibre, which further slows absorption.

Sugar content in fruit increases as it ripens so that very ripe fruit may trigger reactions similar to those caused by refined sugar. I'm not suggesting you eat belly-achers instead of ripe apples but it is best to avoid overly ripe fruit. Another tip, if you find that fruit or juices taken separately cause hypoglycaemic-type symptoms, is to take them ten to fifteen minutes before meals as a starter/aperitif. This way you'll still benefit from the important nutrients in the fruit with-out triggering any erratic changes in the blood glucose level.

The main course that follows the fruit should 'mop up' any troublesome symptoms. Avoid eating fruit with or immediately after meals as this can bring on heartburn and has been known to aggravate hiatus hernia.

Sugar doesn't *cause* diabetes but will aggravate symptoms by throwing blood glucose levels into turmoil. Did you know that, in countries where medical testing of urine isn't

---

Sugar has been linked, of course, to weight problems with the result that many a sweet tooth has turned to artificial sweeteners for support. Unfortunately, researchers suspect, these chemicals may trigger the appetite and make you want to eat more, not less. A bit daft if you've just spent a whole heap of dosh on special diet foods that are supposed to help you lose weight! There is also mounting anecdotal evidence concerning a long list of side-effects. Sweeteners are, of course, regarded as a completely safe food additive. However, some health experts are concerned that, despite ongoing assurances, safety trials were not sufficiently extensive. And since sweeteners turn up in so many foods, it's difficult to avoid them and easy to consume large quantities without realizing it.

---

available, suspected diabetes is diagnosed in the following way. The patient empties his or her bladder near the base of a tree trunk. If ants or other sugar-loving insects congregate quickly, the urine obviously contains sugar! Simple!

Sugar-coated breakfast cereals are obviously very sweet-tasting and many are highly refined. But do you know to what extent? Several brands can be as much as 50 per cent sugar. Put this into context by imagining a bowl half-filled with sugar and then topped up with plain cereal. Even apparently healthy high-fibre breakfast cereals can contain large amounts of hidden sugar. Again, if you're unsure, check the labels.

Whether or not sugar is linked to hyperactivity in children is still unproven but evidence from parents suggests that it is a factor, along with other potential allergens such as food colourings, yeast, corn, and cow's milk. My experience with patients has often found hyperactivity coupled to hypoglycaemia.

Research suggests that it is probably not sugar on its own that provokes or stimulates; sugar water, for example, can have a calming effect. Perhaps it's simply that sugar turns up in foods that do cause problems, triggering hyperactive behaviour when mixed with other risk foods.

There is also accumulating evidence that sugar when combined with fat may be more detrimental to health (e.g. in heart and artery disease) than when eaten alone. A whole variety of foods (biscuits, cakes, sticky buns, chocolate, etc.) contain both. Whatever the case, my own clinic work suggests that it's far healthier to cut right back on sugar. If you need sweetening up, choose cold-pressed raw organic honey, real maple syrup, or blackstrap molasses.

Don't forget: If you have a tendency to cravings or blood sugar problems, get into the habit of eating little and often. Smaller, more frequent meals are easier to digest too.

More tips for controlling blood glucose

- Always have breakfast. Going from yesterday dinner time to today lunch without food means you'll be far more likely to experience symptoms of hypoglycaemia, cravings, hollow hunger, and an energy slump.
- The trace minerals chromium and zinc plus vitamins C, E, and B complex are particularly important when it comes to balancing blood sugar. Find all these in a good quality multivitamin/mineral complex.
- If your chosen multi does not contain chromium or has less than 50mcg, it may be worth taking an additional separate supplement of chromium. I have found that a six-month course of between 100mcg and 200mcg a day is about right. Follow the dosage recommendations on the pack and do not exceed the stated dose.
- Essential fatty acids in the form of evening primrose oil or borage oil are also helpful. Take four to six capsules of EPO or two capsules of borage-based GLA for two months, then half the dose for a further four months. Repeat if symptoms return. Information on where to find reliable products is in Chapter 12.
- Try not to go for long periods of time between pit stops. Snacking between meals keeps energy levels up, reduces dramatic swings in blood glucose and, research suggests, may even help to keep cholesterol down! Eating little and often puts less strain on the digestion and burns calories more efficiently so is good practice if you are trying to lose a few pounds.
- If energy lows are a big problem, try increasing the protein content of your diet. It's worth repeating that protein foods can be more sustaining and satisfy the

appetite for longer than carbohydrates. For example, a decent portion of scrambled eggs or bacon or fish at breakfast is likely to sustain you for longer than toast or cereal.

- Don't give up the complex carbohydrates; they're a vitally important part of a healthy diet. Just remember that adding proteins at breakfast or lunch can save you from the hollow emptiness that often hits hard mid-morning or mid-afternoon.

- Make sure the diet includes plenty of fresh vegetable and salad produce and fresh herbs. These foods may not appear to be filling but they provide not only valuable dietary fibre but also many of the vitamins and minerals essential for keeping energy high and blood glucose balanced.

Foods that help

- All kinds of beans
- Any salad foods and vegetables, including broccoli, cauliflower, cabbage, carrots, courgettes, green beans, sweetcorn, artichokes, snow peas, mangetout, onions
- Avocado
- Brown rice
- Cheese
- Free-range eggs
- Fresh fish
- Hummus
- Jacket potatoes
- Nuts and seeds
- Oat cereal
- Oatmeal porridge

- Organically fed lean meat and poultry
- Pasta, especially brown pasta, lentil pasta, and rice pasta
- Quinoa, buckwheat, millet, bulgur
- Rice cakes
- Rye crackers, rye bread, and black rye (pumpernickel)
- Split peas, chickpeas, lentils
- Whole rye crackers
- Yoghurt

Foods that don't

- Any items made predominantly from white flour or sugar, including cakes, buns and biscuits. If you like baked goods, go for the wholegrain varieties and keep sugar content to a minimum
- Fatty and fried foods
- Some take-aways. Avoid those that are very high in fat and devoid of dietary fibre. Indian menus and vegetable pizzas may be a better bet if you need emergency nourishment and are stuck for fast food ideas
- Sprinkling sugar
- Sugary drinks, lemonade, glucose drinks, cola, fruit-flavoured drinks
- Sweets, toffees, glucose tablets

FIVE

Let food be the music of love

$\backsim$

Aphrodisiac, *n*. Humped, grunting animal with matted hair suffering from vertigo.

Anon

When we first fall in love, it seems as if there is time for everything. The jobs that need doing get done. And those that don't? Well, what's it going to matter in a hundred years' time? Then, for some reason, life's realities take us over. We fret if everything isn't 'up together'. The children or the job or the housework or the shopping all take a higher priority than husbands, wives or partners. Meals are a mad rush. The hard day's work that we once approached with such verve and vigour now leaves us so completely shattered that all we want to do at the end of it is sleep. We wonder how we ever found time to talk. And how on earth did we ever summon the stamina to make love for half the night and still feel alive in the morning? What happened to it all?

Now there's not even enough time for a caress, a kind word or a cuddle at the end of an exhausting day. It doesn't necessarily mean that we don't love one another anymore, just that we're too tired – or too busy – or have simply forgotten how to express it.

OK, so not everyone agrees on the importance of sex in a relationship. Evelyn Waugh preferred going to the dentist. Bette Midler wondered, if it came so naturally, why there needed to be so many books on the subject. James Thurber wanted to know if it was necessary at all and Lawrence Durrell thought it boring. A couple of hundred years ago, the Earl of Chesterfield complained that the pleasure was momentary, the position ridiculous and the expense damnable. Of course, you can still be romantic without being physical. Some couples are content to be without the physical passion but there's no getting away from the fact that keeping the romance alive strengthens and perpetuates a relationship.

Stand back and take a look at yours before it grows dim. When was the last time you sent flowers or wrote a love letter or posted a card expressing how you feel, prepared a candlelit dinner together (or for each other) – or planned a picnic in the bedroom?

If you've been feeling faded and jaded of late, it's no wonder that love-making has slipped to the bottom of the list of exciting things to do. But you can change things. One of the first areas to look at is your diet. Yes, I know. You're wondering how food could possibly make any difference to your sex life. Well it can and it does. Here's how.

Food for lovers

To the first true lovers, an apple was the only aphrodisiac they needed. Since then, many an exaggerated claim has been made for a range of foods that are supposed to turn on the passion. Although no one has yet found the ultimate food-stuff that can produce instant ardour to order, it's certainly true that some foods can be stimulating, others definitely soporific, and a few like water for chocolate.

Some we can understand; one or two we might question.

For example, it isn't difficult to see how ginseng, famed for its ability to improve stamina, might have a positive effect on sexual energy, but what about garlic as an aphrodisiac? A definite turn-off for some people – and even more so if only one partner has eaten it! Although some people clearly don't mind. As a colleague of mine put it: 'I have no problem with my fella eating garlic as long as my ophthalmologist and orthodontist don't!' Perhaps garlic's ability to improve circulation and warm up cold hands and feet has something to do with its popularity as a passion-enhancer? Or the fact that garlic contains zinc, a trace mineral known to be important to fertility, growth, and sexual development.

The zinc link

Many foods that are claimed to have aphrodisiac properties are rich in zinc. For example, half a dozen oysters would meet the health department's recommendations on zinc intake for nearly a week!

Highest concentrations of zinc in humans are to be found in the prostate gland and semen. Men with low levels of the mineral in their blood may also have reduced testosterone.

Crab is an excellent source of zinc, so is lobster. But if these are beyond your budget, no worries. There are plenty of other foods to choose from that don't cost the earth.

Foods famed for their aphrodisiac properties

Almonds	Dates	Oysters
Apples	Figs (fresh and dried)	Pawpaw (papaya)
Artichokes	Fresh fish	Peaches
Asparagus	Fresh ginger	Rosemary
Carrots	Fresh herbs	Smoked salmon
Caviar	Ginseng	Strawberries and
Celery	Goat's cheese	cream
Champagne	Grapes	Tomatoes off the
Cherries	Green vegetables	vine
Chestnuts	Honey	Truffles
Chickpeas	Lamb's liver	Turkey
Chocolate	Lobster	Vanilla
Clams	Mango	Venison
Crab	Mussels	Wild salmon
Crayfish	Nectarines	

But do they work?

Many foods that are supposed to double as aphrodisiacs are simply nutritious ingredients prepared in a wholesome but extra special way. Although it's fun to talk in terms of passionate foods, their link with revving up a romance probably has more to do with the general air of contentment and relaxation induced by a tasty meal and the nourishment gained from it than any likelihood of instant or uncontrollable frenzy!

Since food nutrients are vital for the production of energy and of hormones, the nutrient value of food clearly plays an important role in the love department. Foods that sap our energy, take forever to digest, make us windy, or send us to sleep are obviously best avoided!

The main points about food for romance are how it affects the senses, how it's prepared, what it looks like on the table, and how it's consumed. If you throw the same old stuff together week after week, eat in a hurry so that you can fall asleep in front of the ten o'clock news and never share the preparation or clearing up with anyone, then it's little wonder that mealtimes have become a boring duty. Or maybe you never arrive home early enough to share a meal with your sweetie-pie, anyway. If that sounds like you, the occasional bedroom picnic (see page 84) could be your salvation!

Don't let your love life degenerate to the point where your dinner is in the dog. Keeping the romance alive perpetuates the passion. And that applies whether you're twenty-eight or eighty, met only last month or have been together for years. It's never too late to start. Just because you don't see lights in the sky every time you kiss, doesn't mean it can't be special.

The only good reason for not wanting to get out of bed should be that you don't want to be parted from the person beside you.

If your sex life leaves you wondering why you bother, it may simply be that you haven't the energy to focus the same amount of interest on bedroom activity as you do on other areas of your life. Here are some ideas.

- Stir things up a bit. Take the initiative. Don't let self-consciousness hold you back. Talk to your partner about your needs and pleasures as well as theirs. Remember that it is all too easy to smash someone's sexual self-esteem by sounding disparaging or disapproving. Don't be critical or angry if things aren't as you would wish. Be clear, complimentary and considerate, and discuss what's missing now that used to make sex in the early days so great. (But never give points out of ten.)

- Learn to relax and make relaxation exercises part of your daily routine. Each day, find a quiet moment and take a slow deep in-breath, allowing air to push your diaphragm down and expand your abdomen. Pause for two seconds. Then exhale slowly, discarding unwanted thoughts, stress and negativity. Repeat for ten in-breaths and ten out-breaths. Close your eyes during this exercise and make a mental picture of somewhere you enjoy being – near a river, on a hill looking down at the fabulous view, by the sea, or, perhaps, in a wood or forest where the sun is filtering through a green canopy.

- Instead of having sex to unwind, try relaxing before making love. Treat your partner to a 'back-stroke' and then let him/her do the same for you. Have your partner lie face down on the bed or other firm surface. Place your hands one on each of his/her shoulders. Press down gently and then, using long sweeping movements, bring your hands inwards to the centre of the back and then down the spine to the buttocks. Sweep outwards to the hips and stroke up the sides of the torso until you reach the shoulders again. Make about ten complete movements. Finish by using a very light touch and

---

Try this energizing exercise, either together or alone. See yourself lying on a deserted beach. Picture fresh clear water rushing to the shore, in through the soles of your feet and circulating throughout your body. See the water as energizing and watch it carry energy to your brain, throat, chest, arms, abdomen, genital area, and buttocks. As the water flows back down through your legs, allow any tiredness to drain away with it. With the next wave, repeat the picture, all the time breathing deeply and steadily.

drawing circles and figures of eight all over your partner's back.

- Are you both as fit as you could be? For example, do either of you take enough exercise? Do you always go for the lift or escalator because you get puffed walking up the stairs? Did you know that impotence and lack of interest in sex is more common in those who are not physically fit. Regular exercise really does help to dissipate exhaustion and increase energy.

- Find out if your partner is feeling well. Just because you live with someone, doesn't always mean that you'll know automatically if their health is below par. If there is some health aspect that worries you, talk to your GP. Don't duck out of a medical check-up just because you or they think you're fussing.

- Make sure that you and your partner are eating properly. In just the same way that what we eat affects our general health and our well-being, it can also make the difference between falling asleep depleted and drained in front of the television or deliciously relaxed in each other's arms. When vitamins and/or minerals fall to below normal levels, sexual desire is one of the first things to fade. From a purely practical point of view, improving our diets makes for good health insurance, amongst other things helping to reduce the risk of cardiovascular disease, enhancing immunity, and protecting us against stress. The All Day Energy Diet is also a healthy way to put some pep into your zip.

- If morning finds you a fatigued and lethargic lump of lead, then it sounds as if you might need to make some general changes to your everyday diet as an important step to improving overall health and well-being. When you feel better in yourself, it's probable you will have more time for your partner. The information on boosting energy (Chapter 3) and on maintaining a healthy weight (Chapter 1) are good places to begin.

- If your love life could do with a lift, the ideas in this chapter could give it the excitement it needs. And it isn't necessary to stretch to caviar and champagne or lobster and truffles to make the grade in romantic dining. The recipes in Part 4 are not only good for you, quick to prepare (and fun to do together), but also within sensible shopping budgets. If you want something a little more exotic — and to hell with the calories or the cost — check out the ideas on page 173.

For that memorable night

- Look upon romantic dinners (or days) as extra special and treat them as you would a restaurant meal or rendezvous away from home. Make the effort to dress for dinner. Not only will you look great, you never know when the opportunity might arise to linger longer later over the delicious unzipping and un-buttoning. Allow time for hair, make-up, manicure, pedicure, and perfume.
- Plan your menu well in advance but try to shop on the day or, at least, no earlier than the day before your hot date.
- Go for items that are not part of your everyday shopping list but avoid anything you've never prepared before. Concocting a complicated recipe that hasn't been tried and tested in your own kitchen and flops at the crucial moment can be courting disaster.
- Choose foods that are quick to prepare, easy to serve, and that won't take all night to wash up. Standing at the kitchen sink scouring the soufflé dish will not add to your fascination. Nor will a pile of unwashed pots at breakfast time.

- If you are genuinely short on time or hate cooking, don't be afraid to go for good quality pre-prepared meals. There is a world of difference between junk food and superior fast food. You'll pay more per serving than you would for a regular every-day meal but far less than it would cost in a restaurant. It'll save you time *and* reduce the anxiety of 'getting it right on the night'. You don't have to be a confident cook to succeed at romantic dinners. Search the deli counter in your upmarket supermarket or look round your local delicatessen for ideas.
- Knock tobacco, curry, cucumber, radishes, and beans off the shopping list. Not surprisingly, they are all definite turn-offs in the lovemaking department!
- Avoid the temptation to prepare too much food. A main course and dessert should suffice or, if you don't have a sweet tooth, a starter and main dish. Overeating is a definite *an*aphrodisiac.
- If you're fazed by having to prepare an actual meal, why not go for finger food. It isn't just for kids. Doing without the cutlery can be incredibly sensual (and it saves on the washing up!). Finger food is good to share across the dining table but also terrific fun for bedroom picnics. Page 86 has plenty of suggestions!

The benefits of bedroom picnics

Eating in the boudoir is like camping out in style. Great if you've been to drinks or to the theatre and haven't eaten. Or you've had to work late. Or just anytime you don't feel like slaving over a hot stove or want to put your feet up. Or the kids are sleeping over with friends. It might just be for an evening or a longer night. Decadent Sunday breakfasts in bed or long weekends can be even more fun.

- *Don't* do it in a heat wave unless you have air conditioning. Definitely *do it* in the winter when headline news tells you not to travel unless your journey is absolutely necessary.
- Or when the wind is blowing at gale force or the rain is coming down in stair rods.
- Or any time you feel like a change.

Here's how to plan it:

- If you're lucky enough to have a TV/video or hi-fi set up in the room, organize a romantic film or CD and have it ready to roll as soon as the food is served.
- Coloured nightlights or floating candles enhance the atmosphere. Blue candles stand for serenity, tranquillity, and calmness. Red candles signify sexuality, stimulation, and passion. Pink is best for encouraging tenderness and gentleness.
- Spray your favourite perfume or aftershave on the bedlinen. A couple of squirts should be enough. Overdo it and you could be overwhelmed with scent rather than sensuousness!
- Arrange plenty of pillows and cushions so that you can be really comfortable.
- Clear the bedside table or dressing table of clutter to allow plenty of room for tapes, CDs, books, magazines, and anything else that you think you might need.
- Spread a large tablecloth (or bathtowel) over the bed to protect against accidental spillage.
- Forget the evening gown, girls, and go for sexy underwear or floating negligee. Guys – ditch the vest and boxer shorts and turn up in something tighter.
- Cold food is best – no burnt tongues and no after-dinner

cooking smells in the bedroom. See Tasty Titbits below for ideas.

- Prepare the food on small decorative dishes with a paper napkin to accompany each one. Fingers can get sticky!
- When you choose the wine, remember that white is safer than red in bed. A wine cooler or ice bucket is a nice touch.
- If you don't have pukka wine glasses, it really is worth investing in a pair. They don't have to be expensive but make all the difference to the moment. Coloured glass makes a nice change and will pick up the flickering light from the candles.
- A final tip. Never doubt the turning on talents of toothpaste. However much you enjoyed your sexy dinner, very few lovers like bad breath. And if you wake up to love in the morning, nip to the bathroom and freshen up first.

Eating in bed is one of the greatest pleasures, especially if the refrigerator is full and you have plenty of choice. Even if you're not sharing a relationship with anyone, don't deny yourself the pleasures of a bedroom picnic. Favourite food accompanied by a great film, absorbing novel or relaxing music is still thoroughly enjoyable *tout seul*.

Tasty titbits

- *Asparagus spears.* Cook, drain, douse in butter, and leave to go cold. A good source of most minerals (including zinc!) plus Vitamins C and E and folic acid.
- *Globe artichokes.* Cook, drain, separate the leaves, allow to

go cold and serve with mayonnaise or fresh dressing. Another folic acid-rich vegetable that also contains some zinc.

- *Large prawns.* Yet more zinc plus a good dose of four other important minerals: magnesium, calcium and iron and selenium.

- *Tiny rolls of smoked salmon.* High in sodium, of course, but not something you eat every day. Perhaps not to be recommended if you suffer from raging blood pressure! On the plus side, smoked salmon scores well for potassium and magnesium, two minerals that are good for hypertension. Make the salmon into something really tasty by adding curd cheese and spinach. Buy fresh young spinach, remove any stalks and blanch a few leaves in boiling water for no more than thirty seconds. Run the spinach under cold water and put to one side. Spread each smoked salmon fillet with the curd cheese, roll up, and wrap the outside of each one with a layer of spinach leaves. Wrap tightly in clingfilm and pop into the refrigerator. When you unwrap them, you'll find that they stay together.

- *Cherry (or baby) tomatoes.* For best flavour, stick to summer tomatoes and buy local organic ones if you can (try local nurseries, farms, etc.). Wash them well, eat them whole, dipped into taramasalata. Tomatoes, also called 'love apples', have small amounts of most minerals but are especially good for potassium, carotene, flavonoids, folic acid, and the newly discovered lycopene. They also provide worthwhile dietary fibre. Steer clear of the forced cold-weather varieties that are hard as bullets, picked green and gas-ripened in huge trucks on the way to market. Be aware that some tomato types are now ripening to order as a result of genetic engineering!

- *Mini sticks of chopped celery and carrot* in a favourite dip. These two together will give not only valuable dietary fibre but carotene, zinc, potassium, iron, magnesium, selenium, vitamin C, folic acid, and small quantities of most B vitamins.
- *Slices of chicken breast.* For less hassle, buy breast off the bone (free-range, organically fed if possible). Sauté gently in a little extra virgin olive oil for fifteen minutes, turning the meat several times during cooking. Then allow to cool in the refrigerator. Slice and serve with green salad leaves, tomatoes, and a dip. Chicken is a first-class protein and provider of a range of goodies including iron, zinc, magnesium, selenium, vitamins B3 and B5, plus folic acid. Avoid battery-raised and barn-raised fowl.
- *Bite-sized squares of real cheese.* Another good protein and well known for its ability to keep us awake! Excellent source of calcium, vitamin A, and zinc. Choose fresh (not shrink-wrapped) goat's or sheep's cheeses. Good delicatessens usually have a better range than most supermarkets. Cow's milk cheese can bring out the zits in those with sensitive skin and is also difficult for some people to digest. For those who adore cheese but have difficulty dealing with it, try eating it with fresh pineapple which has natural enzymes to aid digestion.
- *Baby new potatoes.* Choose organic potatoes, wash and boil them with fresh mint, drain, douse with butter and chopped chives. Leave to cool. Or bring new meaning to the phrase 'hot potato' and serve them, just cooked, off the end of a fork, dipped with sour cream. Potatoes are very nutritious, containing vitamin C, B6, potassium, and, if you eat the skin, first-rate dietary fibre.
- *Cheese and Tomato Crumpet* (see page 152). If you are really

hungry and need something hot, this pizza-like snack is an ideal filler.

Dizzy desserts

- *Strawberries*, dipped in sugar and dunked in thick cream. A bedroom picnic is essential during the all-too-fleeting (UK) strawberry season. If you live in a climate where they're available all year, take advantage on special nights! Strawberries have been called the 'best of berries'. They are certainly one of the best sources of vitamin C (seven or eight berries providing more than a whole orange), potassium and some fibre.
- *Seedless grapes*. Great mouth fresheners and another potassium-rich fruit, grapes also provide some calcium, magnesium, and carotene. One of the best 'internal cleansers'.
- *Chunks of pineapple* (helps the digestion). Go for broke and buy a fresh one.
- *Fresh fruit fool*. Take two pieces of any ripe fruit (kiwi, peach, nectarine, mango, pear or banana all work well) and liquidize together with 1 tablespoon of double cream, 2 tablespoons of sheep's yoghurt, 1 teaspoon of cold-pressed liquid honey, and 1 teaspoon of your favourite sherry. Serve in sundae glasses and sprinkle the top with flaked almonds.
- *Fresh creamy yoghurt*. An easy-to-digest protein providing superb calcium scores plus zinc, magnesium, potassium, vitamin A and B vitamins. Make it extra special by stirring in a couple of teaspoons of raw, cold pressed honey – great for licking off the spoon and anywhere else that takes your fancy!

SIX

Supporting the system with supplements

༄

FOR ENERGY

FOR DIETERS

FOR SMOKERS

FOR STRESS

WHAT TO TAKE

HOW MUCH TO TAKE

༄

> There is only about one chance in ten that (a person) will consume the optimum combination and amount of antioxidant (nutrients) on any given day.
>
> Dr Lester Parker, Department of Molecular and Cell Biology, University of California Berkeley

There was a time when I was convinced that vitamin and mineral supplements were unnecessary in most cases. My work with patients over the past ten years has convinced me that this is no longer the case. In fact, anyone who still believes that we can get all the nourishment we need from food alone is probably living in some kind of pollution-free cuckoo land.

The bad news

There is no getting away from the fact that, in one way or another, the food supply is degenerating. Artificial chemicals, fertilizers, herbicides, pesticides, fungicides, toxic waste from industry, traffic exhausts, smoking, radiation, irradiation, genetic engineering, intensive agriculture, factory farming, over-production, preservatives, colourings, flavourings, and other enhancers, long-term storage of produce and extended shelf-life, rushed and hurried eating habits – these are just a few ingredients in the increasingly frightening cocktail that conspires to reduce the nutrient value of our food intake.

It could get you down if you let it.

Yes, we can recycle glass and cardboard, go to work on a bike, boycott beef, and refuse to buy bleached babywear but we have no direct control over the air we breathe.

No one today is able to live in a totally unpolluted, stress-free environment, avoiding all processed food and consuming only organic produce. Even those who are managing to eat the healthiest possible diet can't avoid the stresses, strains, and contaminants that make up modern living. Apart from the fact that very few of us manage to achieve anything like an ideal food intake, most of us are plagued with worries, anxieties, lethargy, exhaustion, and sleep problems. We have too much to do, never enough hours in the day to do it, too many people putting pressure on us, and no time to spare to look after ourselves. We grab meals on the run or sit down only long enough to clear our plates. Our whole existence is one big timetable of 'must do', 'have to'. And most of it happens while we are generally under par.

Think about all the people you know and ask yourself how

many of them have no health problems, are completely fit, have the perfect weight, and are brimming with energy? Hardly any, I bet. Colds are commonplace, weight problems permanent, exhaustion ubiquitous!

The good news

All is far from lost. Making small but significant changes to what we eat and the way we eat it – and adding a very basic but top-quality supplement programme to our daily food supply – can make an enormous difference to how we feel, to our general health and to our stamina. We cope far better when we are properly nourished; energy levels are sustained, we resist infection, sleep better, and wake up wanting to get on with the day instead of longing to go back to sleep.

No need for megadoses

You'll probably have read many articles or books extolling the virtues of a whole range of vitamins and minerals. When you go into pharmacies or health-food stores and see shelf upon shelf groaning under the huge assortment of different brands, I'd be surprised if you didn't end up feeling really confused.

- Which ones are best for you?
- Should you take them all?
- What sort of dosage?
- With food or without?

First of all, there is no need at all to take lots of different tablets or capsules. But there are a few general guidelines which should help you to choose wisely.

The vast majority of vitamin, mineral and other supplements are manufactured to a very high standard. To a great extent, supplement quality is determined by price. In other words, you get what you pay for. Quality products tend to be more bio-available (better absorbed and utilized by the body) than cheaper products. And the more expensive brands are likely to have been subjected to extensive research, development and testing. In other words, buying the *least* expensive brand may be a false economy.

So, go for the best that you can afford. Ask in your health food store for advice. The helplines listed in Chapter 12 can provide information on where to find stockists and, if you can't get to the shops, will tell you how to go about obtaining the best supplements by mail order.

If you have a long-term health problem or are unsure about which products to buy, invest in a consultation with a qualified practitioner who is familiar with the use of nutritional supplements. Details of how to find a therapist are provided in Chapter 12.

Supplements for energy

Even if your diet is near perfect, it's still possible to feel fatigued by work pressure, family commitments, travelling, and lack of sleep. Supplements can give support here too.

Busy Bs

A major player in the energy-boosting team is the group of vitamins known as the B complex. It includes thiamine (vitamin B1), riboflavin (vitamin B2), nicotinic acid (vitamin B3 – also called niacin), pantothenic acid (vitamin B5 – pantothenate), pyridoxine or pyridoxal (vitamin B6), cobalamine (vitamin B12), biotin, and folic acid. Related to the B group, although not strictly vitamins, are PABA, pangamic acid, orotic acid, laetrile, choline, and inositol.

B vitamins are vital for so many different body functions, including converting food substances into energy, for the production and repair of body tissues, supporting the nervous system, and helping us to cope with stress. B vitamins also play an important part in the fight against free radicals which can accelerate cell damage and speed up the ageing process (see The Importance of Antioxidants below).

How much to take

One good multivitamin or B complex daily with either breakfast or lunch should be adequate. Don't take them in the evening (anything containing B vits tends to be stimulating and so could keep you awake!) and never on an empty stomach. A worthwhile product should contain at least the first eight nutrients listed (B1, B2, B3, B5, B6, B12, biotin, and folic acid). I have given the full names as well as the 'B' numbers and hope that this information will be helpful when checking labels. A good guide is to go for a brand that contains 25–50mg of each of the main vitamins B1 to B6.

Co-enzyme Q10 for energy

In addition to your B complex or multi complex, take a course of co-enzyme Q10, a vital supplement for anyone bothered by chronic fatigue, lethargy, weight problems, or exhaustion. It is now widely available through pharmacies and health-food stores. If you think the name is difficult to remember, have sympathy with anyone who had to refer to it by its original title of *2,3,dimethoxy-5-methyl-6-decaprenil-1,4-benzoquinone*! No wonder they decided to call it Q10 or vitamin Q for short! And if you ever see it named Quinone or Ubiquinone, that's because it is found in a wide variety of living things, i.e. it is ubiquitous.

Quinone may sound like an artificial chemical but it is, in fact, a naturally occurring vitamin-like substance which was discovered by scientists as recently as 1957. Since then, it has displayed some very special properties indeed. Studies around the world have found Q10 to be valuable in the treatment of high blood pressure, gum disease, elevated cholesterol, coronary heart disease and, most recently, breast cancer.

Q10's role in energy production is particularly important. Every single cell in the human body contains microscopically small power-producing units called mitochondria, which are responsible for transforming sugars and fats from the diet into usable energy. Areas of the body that need to produce more energy than others – for example, the muscles and the heart – have more mitochondria. Quinone (Q10) is one of the most important nutrients needed by these 'power units' for energy production and, literally, puts fire into the furnace. One scientist likened it to 'pouring petrol on dying embers'. Useful to know if you are suffering from overwork and exhaustion.

In addition, quinone acts as an antioxidant, helping to protect the cellular structure and fight free radical damage. Quinone is found in meat, poultry, oily fish, some nuts, green vegetables, soya, and eggs but only in small amounts and not in sufficient quantities to provide therapeutic doses.

For vegetarians, the levels will be lower still since, as you can see from this list, it appears mainly in animal-based produce.

Quinone is recommended if you suffer from:

- Chronic fatigue syndrome
- Exhaustion
- Heart or circulatory disorders
- High cholesterol
- Hypertension
- Overwork
- Palpitations
- Periodontal (gum) disease
- Stress
- Weight problems
- Also helpful for anyone who undertakes strenuous exercise or is involved in regular sporting activities.

Important note: If you are taking cholesterol-lowering drugs (statins), talk to your GP or pharmacist about taking quinone. They may recognize it by one or all of its other names including co-enzyme Q10 or Vitamin Q. Research suggests that statins may trigger co-enzyme Q10 deficiency, making the need for supplements a strong possibility.

How much to take

Quinone can be expensive but my experience has been that quality really counts. I have found that two 30mg capsules per day are an optimum dose for me. For antioxidant protection and to keep my energy levels high, I take them for six months of the year from October to April but also top them up in summer if I'm travelling abroad or have a heavy schedule – so that means that I take them most of the time! You may find that one capsule daily is sufficient; however, studies show that less than 30mg does not raise blood levels significantly enough to make a difference. In the treatment of cardiomyopathy and other heart conditions or for breast cancer, higher doses are likely to be necessary.

For best absorption, always take your supplement with a main meal (preferably breakfast or lunch, not with dinner). For more information in the UK, ring 0800 591756, 01670 519989 or 0121 433 3727. Technical data and research material is available to pharmacists and other health professionals.

If you are tired all the time and just don't know how you are going to get through the day, treat yourself to a six-month course of B complex (or good multi complex) together with co-enzyme Q10.

The importance of antioxidants

Antioxidants are nutrients that help to protect cells from attack by harmful substances known as free radicals. Free radicals occur naturally in the body but, without antioxidants to keep them in check, can get out of hand.

A low intake of antioxidants and high levels of free radical activity have been linked to premature ageing and to degenerative illnesses such as cancer, heart disease, pancreatitis, arthritis, senile dementia, cataracts, thrombosis, and atherosclerosis. Free radicals wrinkle our skin, age our internal organs, and addle our brains. Over the past decade, more than 6,000 scientific and medical papers have been published on free radicals and antioxidants. Results confirm not only that antioxidant supplements are capable of fighting bio-logical ageing but that people who have a high intake of antioxidant nutrients have less risk of contracting certain types of cancer.

A very interesting study carried out with the help of nurs-ing home residents showed that those who were given antioxidant supplements displayed improved memory and recall, stronger intellectual and emotional ability, and better motor skills.

Ensuring a high intake of antioxidants is important for everyone, especially those working in a polluted environ-ment, breathing in traffic fumes, etc., and for smokers, since inhalation of cigarettes (either directly or passively) creates huge quantities of damaging free radicals.

How much to take

Take one daily antioxidant with breakfast or lunch. The best known antioxidant nutrients are vitamins A, C, E, and the trace mineral selenium. There are many products on the market made up of just these ingredients. However, other vitamins and minerals (vitamins B1, B3, B5, and B6, manganese, and zinc) also play a vital role in the war against free radical damage. The better quality antioxidant supplements are likely, therefore, to contain a wider selection of nutrients but are likely to be more expensive. (See Chapter 12.)

Omega 3 oils

Most of us have read reports that fish oils may be helpful in the fight against heart disease. But they may have value for smokers as well as those with asthma and respiratory allergies too.

If you're a smoker, you'll already know that the best way to prevent damage to the lungs is give it up. However, protection is still important while you are cutting down or giving up (and especially so if quitting is not an option). New research shows that a daily intake of Omega 3 essential fatty acids (found predominantly in fish oil and nutritional grade linseed oil) can improve lung capacity and help to reduce the risk of chronic obstructive pulmonary diseases (COPD) such as emphysema and bronchitis. Studies show that the anti-inflammatory properties of these therapeutic oils are able to reduce wheezing and breathing difficulties as well as joint pain and stiffness, making them useful in reducing the symptoms of asthma and allergies, and valuable in soothing the pain of arthritis. I have also seen patients suffering from the troublesome skin condition, psoriasis, benefit from daily fish oil supplements. Fish oil is also used to treat hypertension (high blood pressure) and is available in the UK on prescription for this condition.

How much to take

Studies show that people who eat oily fish two or three times per week do not normally need to take fish oil capsules as well. However, I have found that patients suffering with obstructive airway disease, asthma, hayfever and other allergies, do benefit from a one-daily supplement of fish oil. Choose capsules that provide around 1000mg per day. If you are vegetarian, or for some other reason are unable to eat fish or take fish oil capsules, then go for 1000mg of linseed oil. Chapter 12 has details of where to find specialist products.

Important note: The polyunsaturated fatty acids in fish oil can, unfortunately, turn rancid (oxidise) extremely easily. Taking a quality antioxidant supplement with fish oil can help to reduce the risk of damage to the oils and consequent free radical activity.

Good sources of fish oil		
Cod	Fresh and canned	Seafood
Flatfish	sardines	Sprats
Fresh and canned	Halibut	Trout
mackerel	Herring	Tuna
Fresh and canned	Mussels	Whitebait
salmon	Oysters	

Vitamin C

A major anti-stress vitamin and an absolutely vital antioxidant that works closely with vitamin E and selenium to counteract the harmful effects of oxidation. All antioxidant supplements should contain reasonable amounts of Vitamin C. However, some experts are now convinced that the official recommendation of 40–60mg per day from diet is woefully inadequate. Worryingly, many sectors of the population do not eat enough fresh produce even to achieve this small intake. It has been estimated that one cigarette or a few lungfuls of polluted air can use up 25mg of vitamin C. In fact, smokers and passive smokers need more than twice the amount of vitamin C as non-smokers who avoid the pollutant altogether, since the free radicals initiated by the chemicals in cigarettes use up large quantities of this vitamin. Stress also swallows up massive quantities of vitamin C.

If you're plagued by lethargy or stress, it's worth knowing that vitamin C plays a major role in supporting the nervous system and in the production of energy. Without it, the body's absorption of iron is reduced. One of the major symptoms of iron deficiency is extreme tiredness.

How much to take

One gram daily (1000mg) of vitamin C if you live/work in a country environment and *do not* suffer from any kind of recurring infections, allergies, or stress. Otherwise, take two grams (2000mg) daily. When choosing vitamin C products, avoid those that contain only ascorbic acid. My experience with patients has been that acidic forms of vitamin C can cause digestive discomfort. Go, instead, for labels which include the words 'low acid', 'buffered', or 'complex' as these are usually kinder to sensitive stomachs. At the recommended levels, they are completely safe and non-toxic.

Note: You may have read some adverse publicity and misinformation that large amounts of vitamin C cause kidney stones. This is a myth that has been around for quite a time and is still bandied about as factual information. It isn't. Despite several scourings of the literature, I have not been able to find any reliable reports or scientific or medical evidence that proves low acid vitamin C complex to be toxic or dangerous even at several grams per day.

If you live or work in a polluted environment, spend time in the town or city, travel for more than an hour a week in heavy traffic, smoke, live or work with smokers, or suffer excessive stress, frequent infections, colds and flu, asthma, or allergies, try this protective supplement programme:

- One daily antioxidant
- Two grams (2000mg) vitamin C complex
- One gram (1000mg) of omega 3 fish oil

These supplements are also recommended to anyone who exercises extensively every day or is involved in regular aerobics or sports activity. For more information on which products to choose, see Chapter 12.

Citrimax (Garcinia cambogia)

If the war against weight loss seems totally lost and you are utterly defeated by the thought of another diet, it could well be worthwhile following a course of Citrimax, a supplement produced from the plant *Garcinia cambogia*. Garcinia is a rich source of a substance known as HCA (hydroxy citric acid) that, research has shown, may be valuable in helping to turn fat into energy and in synthesizing cholesterol. Citrimax Forte is a natural source of the trace minerals manganese and chromium that assist in balancing blood glucose levels, so increasing energy levels and reducing cravings. And vitamin B5 and vitamin C are there to give additional support to the adrenal glands.

Garcinia cambogia is not an appetite suppressant or weight loss drug. It isn't a short-cut to weight reduction; nor is it a substitute for a healthy diet or sensible exercise. However, a course of six to twelve weeks on Citrimax Forte can kick stubborn weight into touch and provide the incentive to stick to a healthy diet. Take one tablet three times daily, thirty minutes to an hour before each meal.

You will need to see your GP or dietician for a check-up

before commencing the course. Suppliers will happily provide technical and research data to health professionals.

Note: Garcinia supplements are not suitable for anyone who suffers migraine or intolerance to citric acid.

Spirulina

Spirulina is a blue-green algae, rich in protective antioxidants and easily digestible protein. It is also a valuable source of vitamin B12, normally found only in animal products and therefore recommended to vegetarians and vegans. A nutrient-rich energy boost for anyone feeling under-par or recovering from illness, spirulina is also recommended to athletes and to sports and fitness enthusiasts. It is available in tablet form but also in powder and flakes. Sprinkle it on to salads and cereals and into soups and stews. Deserves a permanent place on the shopping list. Highly recommended to anyone who has a problem 'eating their greens'! Available from health-food stores or by mail order (see Chapter 12).

Aloe vera juice

Apart from its recorded benefits as a treatment for burns, cuts, grazes, bedsores and all manner of other skin problems, aloe vera is also used as a digestive tonic, reputed to raise energy levels and enhance well-being. Take it daily as a pre-breakfast drink, mixed with your fruit juice if you like. When choosing aloe (and spirulina), buy the best that you can afford, sticking to the general rule that more expensive food supplements tend to be of a higher quality. Stockist details are in Chapter 12.

PART THREE

The All Day Energy Eating Plan

SEVEN

Getting started

ॐ

This chapter should give you plenty of encouragement on your new healthy eating journey. You'll find lots of information on the best foods to choose for energy, a whole variety of vegetable, salad, and snack ideas, delicious fruits, and suggestions on store cupboard items and kitchen equipment to make choosing, preparing, and shopping that much easier.

Energy-boosting ideas

Protein-based foods

Beancurd	Lamb's liver
Buttermilk	Lean lamb
Free-range eggs	Quorn
Free-range poultry	Sheep's milk cheese
Fresh fish	Tofu
Goat's milk cheese	Yoghurt

Starchy foods

Barley	instead of ordinary wheat flour)
Basmati rice	
Brown rice	Buckwheat grains (Kasha)
Buckwheat flour (use	Buckwheat pasta

Bulgur wheat
Couscous
Jacket potatoes (organic
     only)
Matzos
Millet
Muesli (choose wheat-free or
     gluten-free)
Oat biscuits
Oat-based cereals
Oats
Oat bran

Pasta (see page 116)
Porridge
Potato flour (another alter-
     native to wheat flour)
Pumpernickel
Quinoa
Rice cakes
Rice flour
Rye bread
Rye crackers
Sweet potatoes
Wild rice

Useful sweeteners

If you have a sweet tooth, being told to avoid sugar can be a fate almost worse than a fat-free, cholesterol-free, caffeine-free cappuccino. And as I've explained on page 71, artificial sweeteners may not be the answer for everyone. The sweetenings listed below provide healthier alternatives to refined sugar and chemically derived sugar substitutes. However, they should be used in moderation only.

Blackstrap molasses
Carob spread
Crystallized ginger
Fructose powder (fruit

sugar)
Honey – cold-pressed, raw
     organic
Real maple syrup

Good food ideas

Vegetable and salad foods

Aim to eat two or three servings per day chosen from this list, either as freshly cooked vegetables accompanying a main meal, or in salads, soups, stir-fries or casseroles.

Artichokes
Asparagus
Aubergine (eggplant)
Avocado
Bamboo shoots
Beansprouts
Beet greens
Beetroot
Broccoli, green and purple
Brussels sprouts
Cabbage – dark leaf varieties have more nourishment
Calabrese
Capsicums (red, yellow, or green bell peppers)
Carrots (organic only)
Cauliflower
Cauliflower greens
Celeriac
Celery
Chicory
Chives
Courgette (zucchini)

Dandelion greens
Endive
Garlic
Kale
Leek
Lettuce – dark leaf varieties have more nourishment
Mangetout
Marrow
Mushrooms
Mustard & cress
Onion
Shallots
Spinach
Spring onions
Sprouted seeds
Sugar snap peas
Swede (rutabaga)
Tomatoes
Turnip greens
Turnips
Watercress

Culinary herbs

Adding herbs not only improves flavour but also increases the nutritional value of the meal and, in many cases, can help digestion. Most supermarkets now stock growing or freshly cut herbs. Here are a few suggestions.

Basil   Mint
Bay   Oregano
Chives   Parsley
Coriander   Sage
Fennel   Tarragon
Marjoram   Thyme

Fresh fruit

Try to include two or three pieces of fresh fruit each day,
preferably before meals (as a starter) or between meals as a
snack. Eating fruit with a main course or immediately after-
wards as a dessert can disturb digestion in some people. It has
also been found that, where there are weight problems,
eating fruit separately from other food helps to encourage
better absorption of vitamins and minerals. Here are a few
suggestions.

Apples   Kiwi
Apricots   Lemon
Banana   Lime
Blackberries   Mango
Blackcurrants   Melon
Blueberries   Nectarines
Cherries   Papaya
Dried fruit (figs, raisins,   Passionfruit
   sultanas etc.)   Peaches
Figs   Pears
Grapefruit   Pineapple
Grapes   Raspberries
Hunza apricots   Strawberries

Going organic

The All Day Energy Diet recipes take into account the fact that it is not possible for most people to use entirely organic produce at every meal. However, it really is worth going for organic vegetables, organic free-range eggs, etc. whenever you can. Most studies show that fresh organic produce contains more nourishment than its commercially produced counterparts and, of course, no artificial chemicals are used in its production. It also tastes so much better and is not troubled by that strange chemical aftertaste that afflicts so many mass-produced vegetables, salads, and other goods. Organic potatoes, mushrooms, onions, and carrots are all widely available in supermarkets now. If you can't find them, ask for help – or look for a local organic farm (Chapter 12 has details).

When organic alternatives are not available, make sure that vegetables are washed thoroughly and peeled whenever possible. You won't remove all chemicals (the atmosphere is probably too polluted) but should reduce the load. Since reports about heavy pesticide residues in carrots continue to hit the headlines (I find there is a very detectable and unpleasant aftertaste), I would advise avoiding them entirely and buying only organic as and when available. To those who try to assure us that pesticide residues are safe, I always ask 'How can you really tell, when they have been in use for such a relatively short period of time?'

I'd like to have 'P' numbers on produce that is sprayed with pesticides, herbicides, and fungicides – plus openly available safety data – so that we know what goes on to it and into it and can then decide if we want to buy.

A *word about bagged salads*

All supermarkets and a number of grocery stores now stock a wide range of tempting salads in bags, ready washed and sliced or chopped and wonderfully time-saving. It's worth bearing in mind, though, that – once cut into – any vegetable or fruit will lose much of its nutrient content (especially vitamin C) extremely quickly. I also wonder about the preserving process that keeps these ready-to-serve ranges fresh for so many days and how this might affect the level of very important antioxidant nutrients.

Preparing salads at home from scratch is likely to provide more nourishment but only if the ingredients are really fresh and served straight away. Wilting lettuce, wizened capsicums, and warped cucumber will probably be no better for you than ready-to-use salad in bags. Making your own may also be more difficult if you live alone or are the only one in the home who eats salad foods. I think the answer is to use very fresh basic ingredients wherever possible and buy the ready-to-eat kinds at other times, bearing in mind that it is probably better to have salad from bags than no salad at all. Up your antioxidant intake by making sure that your diet also contains lots of other freshly prepared vegetable foods.

You can add extra nourishment to any salad by sprinkling it with a spoonful of spirulina flakes and/or pumpkin seeds and sunflower seeds.

In addition, consider taking a daily multivitamin/mineral or antioxidant supplement (see Chapter 6 for more information on this very important subject).

Not so good for you

Don't rely on these foods too often.

- Battery or barn eggs (choose organically fed free-range)
- Battery or barn-raised poultry (choose organically fed free-range)
- Beef (unless organic)
- Bread – some types (see page 37)
- Cheeses that are coloured, smoked or processed
- Chocolate – choose organic
- Coffee/tea – limit to three cups a day maximum, one if possible. If you're a coffee addict, try weaning yourself on to grain-based coffee substitutes such as Caro or Bambu
- Cow's milk – use in tea or coffee only (see page 34)
- Diet drinks
- Diet foods
- Fizzy drinks, e.g. cola
- Hydrogenated vegetable oils (check labels)
- Ice-cream
- Low-fat foods that contain large numbers of additives
- Margarine spreads
- Oranges and orange juice
- Peanuts
- Pork (unless organic)
- Refined white flour
- Salt and salty foods
- Sugar
- Sugar-coated breakfast cereals
- Wheat-based breakfasts

Swap shop

Help boost your energy and nutrient reserves by eating less of the items in column A and more of those in column B.

A	B
Deep-fried foods	Grill, bake, casserole, steam, stir-fry, or wok it instead
Ordinary cooking oils	Extra virgin olive oil
Margarine or low-fat spreads	Butter or non-hydrogenated spread
Crisps, peanuts, and other salted snacks	Almonds, brazils, hazelnuts, macadamias, pecans, walnuts, sunflower seeds, pumpkin seeds
Sweets, cakes, and doughnuts	Wholegrain cereal bars, natural liquorice, dried fruits, fresh fruit
Ordinary chocolate	Organic chocolate (it's delicious)
Packaged orange juice	Apple or grape juice, or buy a juicer and make your own
Coffee, tea, and cola	Savoury beverages, water, fresh fruit juice, vegetable juice, herbal or fruit teas, soup
Foods full of additives	Foods that aren't!
Battery or barn-raised poultry and eggs	Organic/free-range poultry and eggs
Wheat-based or sugar-coated cereal	Oat porridge, gluten-free muesli

Cow's milk	Soya milk or almond milk*
Cow's milk cheeses	Sheep's or goat's cheese
Ordinary mass-produced bread	Yeast-free soda bread, pumpernickel, rye, rice cakes, oat biscuits, matzos, pittas
Beef or pork	Fresh fish (especially the oily kinds), lean lamb, lamb's liver, free-range organic poultry
Convenience meals and take-aways	Prepare more of your own from fresh basic ingredients so that you know what goes into them

* How to make almond milk: Place ten blanched almonds in a liquidizer with ¼ pint (125ml) of water and blend until you have a smooth 'milk'. Dilute with more water if desired. The mixture will stay fresh in the refrigerator for twenty-four hours and can be stirred into cereal, desserts, yoghurt, and coffee.

Store cupboard essentials

- *Cold-pressed raw organic dark liquid honey*. Good quality honey will cost more. As a general guide in the UK, I would say that anything less than £1.50 per jar is probably not the best quality. There are a few cheaper brands of organic honey on the market but these are not always cold pressed. Once heat treated, any goodness will be destroyed. I use Raw Manuka Honey from New Zealand. If you're confused by the different brands available, ask your health-food store for advice. See Chapter 12 for supplier information.
- *Extra virgin olive oil*. For cooking and salad dressings.
- *Bambu* – organic grain/chicory powder. Good alternative

if you are trying to cut down on coffee. Best taken black.

- *Buckwheat flour and potato flour.* Gluten-free alternatives to ordinary wheat flour. Potato flour is useful for gravies and sauces. Buckwheat makes first-class pancakes. The dark colour of buckwheat can make it look a bit like cement mix but I find the flavour is excellent.
- *Brown rice.* A staple stand-by. Good for adding to so many different dishes – hot or cold.
- *A choice of dried pasta.* Try organic spelt, kamut, rice, rice & ginseng, rye, or legume pasta; all should be available (or can be ordered) from your local health-food store. Spelt and kamut are cultivated from ancient wheat grains untouched by modern agricultural hybridization and grown organically under the strictest regulations. It has been my experience that they are well tolerated even by those who suffer from wheat intolerance. However, if you are unsure, test by trying only very small amounts to begin with. All these pastas provide superior taste and excellent nourishment. They all come in a variety of shapes and sizes from straight spaghetti to vermicelli (birds' nests), fettuccine and tagliatelle (ribbon strips), conchiglie (shells), and fusilli (twists). Rice and legume pastas are suitable for those on wheat-free and gluten-free diets.

Other nourishing foods to try

- Lentils
- Oat bran (makes great porridge)
- Rice cakes
- Rye crackers
- Spirulina (see page 103)
- Aloe vera juice (see page 103)

Nibbles

Nuts and seeds figure prominently in The All Day Energy recipes but, together with dried fruit, they're also valuable as snacks and nibbles. Try these – on their own or mixed in any combination.

- Brazils
- Dried figs
- Flaked almonds
- Linseeds
- Organic dried fruit
- Pine nuts
- Pumpkin seeds
- Sunflower seeds
- Unblanched almonds
- Walnuts or pecans

Cans

- Aduki beans
- Black-eyed beans
- Cannellini beans
- Chickpeas
- Pinto beans
- Red kidney beans
- Mixed pulses

If you have time to prepare dried beans in advance, so much the better. However, canned beans are a good alternative as long as you remember to tip the contents into a sieve and rinse away the salty/sugary liquid that comes with them.

- Baked beans in tomato sauce (original, not low-cal)
- Sardines (best in water, second best in brine, third choice in olive oil, fourth choice in vegetable oil)
- Pink salmon (not as expensive as red and just as good)

For added flavour

In an ideal world, the best seasoning comes from fresh ingredients; i.e. fresh herbs, fresh ginger, fresh pesto, parmesan grated off the block, tomatoes off the vine, etc. The fresher the ingredients, the more nourishment to be had from them, too.

Unfortunately, it isn't always possible to have such luxury to hand, especially if you don't live close to the shops, are stuck for transport or have to rely on someone else to shop for you. The answer is to choose fresh alternatives wherever possible and to use good quality storecupboard stand-bys at other times.

Mixed dried herbs

I pick and dry fresh herbs from the garden during the summer months and store them for winter use. Or pop fresh leaves into an ice-cube tray, top up with filtered water, and freeze for later. When they all run out, I turn to Italian Seasoning or the range of flavourings from Bioforce (Chapter 12).

Other useful flavourings are:

- Balsamic vinegar
- Beetroot in red wine

- Cider vinegar
- English mustard
- Ground ginger
- Herb salt such as Trocamare or Herbamare
- Molkosan (see page 172)
- Organic vegetable stock powder, paste, or cubes – apart from being useful for cooking, they make delicious savoury drinks
- Pesto sauce
- Soy sauce
- Sun-dried tomatoes in olive oil

Useful kitchen equipment

- Water filter jug. The improved quality and taste of the water should encourage you to drink more fluid. It certainly raises tea and coffee into a different class. If you have a jug filter, change the cartridge once a month. Use filtered water for drinking, making tea and coffee, and for cooking.
- Coffee grinder. Great for grinding up pumpkin seeds, sunflower seeds, and linseeds.
- Food processor/blender. Invaluable, especially for soups and desserts. Buy one with vegetable slicing attachments to make light work of coleslaw, onions for sauces, crudités, etc.
- Juicing machine. Makes wonderful juices from fresh fruit and vegetables, which are an important part of The All Day Energy Diet plan.

For most of the items in this chapter, your local health-food shop is the best place to start shopping. Water filter jugs and replacement cartridges are also available from hardware stores, pharmacies, and chemist chains. Coffee grinders (to grind your seeds), juicers, and blenders can be obtained from electrical stores. Extra virgin olive oil can be found in health-food stores and all major supermarkets. Refer to Chapter 12 for details of suppliers.

My thanks to the Kenwood Company for supplying the Jug Blender, Hand Blender and Juicer which were used in the preparation of All Day Energy recipes.

EIGHT

Where to begin

ᔥ

Impossibilium nulla obligatio est
[There is no legal obligation to perform impossibilities]
Aulus Cornelius Celsus

Week one

WEEK ONE is PREPARATION WEEK, helping you to get into some healthier eating habits before you begin the full diet in seven days time. Put your plan into action by following the twelve points listed below.

1   Starting tomorrow, aim to get up just a quarter of an hour earlier than usual. If you normally rise at 7.30am, fall out at 7.15. If you're an earlier bird at 7.00am, then make it 6.45 instead. That special fifteen minutes gives you extra breathing space and reduces the stress and panic that so often goes with getting up in the morning. Being more relaxed and under less pressure are both important parts of your new healthy eating plan.

2   Before showering or bathing, drink a glass of water, filtered or bottled, but not directly from the tap. See my note about water filters on page 119. Or a glass of fresh juice with added aloe vera (see page 103). Increasing

your fluid intake not only lifts energy levels by freshening the system and helping the kidneys to function more efficiently but also improves digestion and elimination. Extra fluid is important during hot weather and during colder spells, preventing dehydration, improving blood volume and reducing the risk of strokes and heart attacks. Keep up your improved fluid intake by drinking another glass of water at about 10am and a further one at about 3pm; that's in addition to your normal intake of other fluids. Carry on with the good habit when you begin the diet next week.

3   With the first fluid of the day, take two capsules of acidophilus (Blackmores, Natran or Biocare) and a 20ml measure of Bioforce Molkosan. Both these products help to improve the general functioning of the digestive system by making it a more favourable environment for beneficial gut bacteria. Do this from now on, throughout the diet, and for a total of three months. Chapter 12 has details of where to find products.

4   This week, make a real effort to cut down on the Not So Good For You foods listed in Chapter 7. Don't lose sleep if you can't avoid them all. Just do what you can. In particular, reduce coffee intake slowly throughout the week so that you are taking only one cup per day by next Sunday! No, you don't have to give up coffee forever but it will be helpful to drink less of it, especially for the duration of The All Day Energy Eating Plan. As an alternative, try grain-based coffee substitutes such as Bambu or Caro (best taken black), fresh fruit juices, water, soups, and savoury drinks (see page 112).

5   Buy extra fruit during this first week and eat more of it.

Choose any fresh fruit (except oranges). Aim for three pieces per day either before or between meals; for example, one before your main breakfast, one sometime during the morning and another in the afternoon.

6 Try to eat more salad and more vegetables too. Instead of ordering chips, have a side salad with the main course. Or ask for extra green vegetables.

7 Everyone has individual tastes and food preferences so, before you begin, read through the recipes, and make a note against the ones you want to use. Don't dismiss out of hand any foods you are not so familiar with. Try them first.

8 If you haven't already done so, turn to Chapter 7. Study the Good for You list and make sure that you have at least the basic items in your store cupboard and refrigerator for the recipes you are choosing.

9 Then look at the Daily Meal Planner at the beginning of Part 4. You'll find fourteen days of nourishing and energizing breakfasts, lunches, and dinners. After you have completed the Week One Preparation, follow the Daily Meal Planner for the next two weeks. It may be that you decide you'll stay with only one or two breakfasts throughout the week rather than have a different one each day. That's fine. The whole point about eating The All Day Energy way is that breakfast should be substantial and not leave you feeling empty by eleven o'clock. The choices really are up to you. It's possible that you aren't able to stop at lunchtime every day to prepare a hot meal. In that case, you may find it easier to go for those lunch suggestions that can be prepared the night before and are easily transportable.

10 When you first begin to use the recipes, I think you'll find it easier to follow the Daily Meal Planner.

However, when you are familiar with the basics, you may decide to turn directly to the recipe sections themselves and choose your own individual preferences.

11 Providing that you are taking regular exercise while you are following The All Day Energy Diet, you should be feeling more active and energized after a week or so. If you are using the Diet to help you lose weight, expect to see slow and steady weight loss by the end of week three. If you have more weight to lose, repeat weeks two and three, alternating and adjusting the recipes to suit your own schedule. Aim to lose no more than a kilo every seven days. Losing weight quickly may seem like a good idea but is likely to result in rapid weight gain later on.

12 **The All Day Energy Diet is not designed as a short-term quick fix programme but is intended as a guide to eating healthily and sensibly in the long term. When you have followed the plan for three weeks, resolve to fit at least some of the healthy eating suggestions into your daily routine. Return to the Diet any time you feel you are lacking energy or slipping back into those not-so-good habits!**

The Entertaining Dinners are not included in the Daily Meal Planner. I'll leave it to you to turn to them when there is a special occasion or lazy weekend in the offing (Chapter 11). Don't forget to enjoy the Tasty Titbits on page 86, too.

Weeks two and three

After seven days of preparation, you are now ready to begin The All Day Energy Diet proper. Part 4 of this book is packed with healthy, delicious, and simple to prepare recipes for Sustaining Breakfasts (Chapter 9), Quick and Easy Lunches and Simple Suppers (Chapter 10), and Easy Entertaining (Chapter 11). At the start of Part 4 you will find the Daily Meal Planner, a quick-reference suggested menu for breakfast, lunch and supper for each of the fourteen days of this stage of The All Day Energy Diet.

Remember to refer back to Chapter 6 for details on supplements, and to Chapter 7 for lists of foods that are good (and bad) for you. If you have difficulty getting hold of any of the ingredients or supplements, refer to Chapter 12.

PART FOUR

Recipes

꒰

There is no love sincerer than the love of food.
George Bernard Shaw, *Man and Superman*

V Recipes marked with this symbol are suitable for vegetarians.

Essential weights and measures

1 tablespoon		15ml
1 dessertspoon		10ml
1 teaspoon		5ml
1 cup	8fl.oz	225ml
	1fl. oz	28ml
1 pint	20fl. oz	570ml
½ pint	10fl. oz	290ml
	1oz	30g
	2oz	55g
	3oz	85g
¼lb	4oz	110g
	7oz	200g
½lb	8oz	225g
1lb	16oz	450g

Daily meal planner

Day	Breakfast	Lunch	Supper
1	Fruit Platter (page 132) and Nut and Seed Yoghurt (page 133)	Chunky Vegetable Soup with rye crackers or naan bread (page 143)	Mixed Vegetable Mozzarella (page 150)
2	Creamy Oat Bran Porridge (page 132)	Crudités with Curd Cheese (page 153)	Sultana Rice and Beans (page 151)
3	Banana Yoghurt Crush (page 134)	Avocado and Rice Tortillas (page 160) or Rainbow Rice (page 156)	Pasta Robusto (page 155) or Egg-fried Rice (page 167)
4	Rice Cakes with Butter and Honey (page 138) or Soda Bread and Honey (page 133)	Quick Can Salad (page 150)	Spicy Vegetable Casserole (page 165) or Bean Bake (page 167)
5	Big Egg Breakfast (page 135)	Easy Leek and Potato Soup served with ciabatta bread or rice cakes (page 152)	Sugar Snap Stir-fry (page 161)
6	Special Recipe Gluten-free Muesli with almond milk (page 136)	Cheese Omelette with Onion and Herbs (page 142) or Matzo Crackers with Avocado and Tomato (page 153)	Vegetarian Minestrone with Penne (page 156)
7	Grilled Bacon with Mushrooms and Tomatoes (page 136) or Scrambled Eggs with Vine Tomatoes (page 139)	Avocado and Hummus Salad (page 142)	Hearty and Healthy Chip Butties (page 158)

Day	Breakfast	Lunch	Supper
8	Rice Cakes with Butter and Honey (page 138) or Yeast-free Soda Bread with Butter and Honey (page 133)	Prawn and Pepper Quick-Fry (page 154)	Simple Pasta with Pesto (page 160)
9	Hunza Apricots with Yoghurt (page 139)	Matzo Crackers with Avocado and Tomato (page 153)	Colourful Veggi Casserole (page 146)
10	Home-made Muesli with almond or soya milk (page 137) or Fruity Yoghurt Cup (page 134)	Jacket Potato; choose from 10 fillings (page 147)	Mixed Vegetable Gratin (page 168)
11	Nut and Seed Yoghurt (page 133)	Thick and Creamy Lentil and Potato Soup with matzo crackers or rice cakes (page 145)	Buckwheat Noodles with Cabbage (page 163)
12	Scrambled Eggs with Vine Tomatoes (page 139)	Wholemeal Pitta Bread; choose your own filling (page 149)	Creamy Cabbage Casserole (page 162)
13	Fruit Platter (page 132) or Hunza Apricots with Yoghurt (page 139)	Cheese and Tomato Crumpet (page 152)	Speedy Gonsalsa (page 159) and Grated Salad Garnish (page 171)
14	Undyed Smoked Haddock with Poached Egg (page 141) or Banana Yoghurt Crush (page 134)	Vegetarian Bolognese (page 164)	Potato Chip Tortillas (page 159) or Avocado and Rice Tortillas (page 160)

NINE

Sustaining breakfasts

❧

V *Fruit Platter*

Choose any fresh fruit in season and make a large serving.

SUGGESTIONS:
1 pear, 1 apple, and 1 small bunch of seedless grapes
1 fresh mango, 1 kiwi fruit, and 1 peach or nectarine
Half a melon with a dozen or so black grapes

V *Creamy Oatbran Porridge (Serves 2)*

3 cups of (cold) filtered water
1 cup of oat bran

OPTIONAL ADDITIONS FOR EACH SERVING:
1 teaspoon of cold-pressed raw liquid honey
2 teaspoons of cream or crème fraîche
1 banana

As porridge saucepans are notoriously unpleasant to clean,
use a non-stick pan for this breakfast.

Pour 3 cups of (cold) filtered water into the pan and add 1
cup of oat bran. (If you try to mix the oat bran with hot or
boiling water, it will go lumpy.)

Stir the cold mixture thoroughly until smooth.

Turn on the heat and bring to the boil, stirring all the time to avoid burning. Simmer until porridge thickens.

Packet instructions usually advise cooking for 2 to 3 minutes. Best cooking time is, in fact, 6 to 8 minutes.

Pour into bowls and serve with a teaspoon of honey, a chopped banana, and 2 teaspoons of cream.

V *Yeast-Free Soda Bread with Butter and Honey*

3 slices of yeast-free soda bread
Butter
Cold-pressed raw honey or sugar-free preserve

Nearly all health-food stores, most supermarkets and some bakeries now stock soda bread. I have already mentioned that some kinds of bread can cause fatigue and drowsiness. Yeast-free soda bread seems to be well tolerated even by those who cannot cope with ordinary wheat-based loaves. However, the only way to find out is to experiment.

V *Nut and Seed Yoghurt*

1 medium carton of goat's milk yoghurt
1 dessertspoon of blanched almonds
1 dessertspoon of walnut or pecan halves
1 dessertspoon of linseeds
1 dessertspoon of cold-pressed raw organic honey

Grind the nuts and seeds and stir them into the yoghurt with the honey.

V *Banana Yoghurt Crush*

1 small carton of sheep's (or goat's) yoghurt
1 dessertspoon of pumpkin seeds
1 dessertspoon of sunflower seeds
1 dessertspoon of seedless raisins or sultanas
1 banana

For a filling breakfast, 8fl. oz (220g) of yoghurt is about right. Sheep's milk yoghurt is smoother and less tart than that made with goat's milk but if only goat's milk yoghurt is available and you find it too sharp, then add a teaspoon of cold-pressed raw honey. Use organic cow's milk yoghurt only if the other types are not available. If the yoghurt label doesn't say what kind of milk has been used, it is almost certainly cow's milk but won't be organic unless labelled.

Crush all the seeds in a coffee grinder. Then put all the ingredients into a blender/liquidizer and mix until smooth. Serve immediately. The point about crushing the seeds is that you will get more goodness out of them that way. However, don't worry if you don't yet have a coffee grinder; use a rolling pin or just put all the ingredients straight into the blender without first crushing the seeds and enjoy a crunchier result!

V *Fruity Yoghurt Cup*

1 medium carton of sheep's or goat's yoghurt
1 small cup of raspberries (for best vitamin value use fresh or frozen; otherwise use canned raspberries in natural juice)
1 ripe kiwi fruit
1 dessertspoon of flaked almonds
1 teaspoon of raw liquid honey

2 teaspoons of organic mixed dried fruit
3 dried figs (chopped)
Half a cup of almond milk (see below)

Mix the dry ingredients together, and pour on the almond milk to serve.

Make the almond milk like this. Blanch a dozen almonds by dousing them in boiling water for a couple of minutes and removing the skins. Then add the nuts to a blender with half a cup of water and mix until you have a fine white liquid.

V *Home-made Muesli*

This is a wheat-free breakfast.

1 dessertspoon of each of the following:
oat bran or oat meal
organic mixed dried fruit
organic dates (chopped)
broken or crushed walnuts or pecans
flaked almonds
pine nuts
linseeds
pumpkin seeds
sunflower seeds
spirulina flakes (see page 103)

3 tablespoons filtered water
1 banana, chopped into small pieces
1 grated carrot (optional)

Note: Buy whole fresh nuts and crush them at home. Nuts that are already broken or crushed when you purchase them are rarely of good quality.

Stir the oats into the filtered water and leave to soak in the refrigerator overnight. In the morning, stir all the remaining ingredients into the oats. The grated carrot is an unusual optional extra that provides colour and extra sweetness. This breakfast should be moist enough to eat without adding milk. If you find the mixture too dry for your taste, add a tablespoon of single cream or a little almond milk (see page 137).

Spirulina flakes are an excellent source of a wide range of vitamins (including B12), minerals, enzymes, carotenes, amino acids, essential fatty acids, chlorophyll, and trace elements.

V *Rice Cakes with Butter and Honey*

This is a useful lightweight breakfast for those who can't face too much food first thing in the morning. It is also portable and so can be taken to work or eaten in the car.

4 rice cakes
Butter or non-hydrogenated vegetable spread
Cold-pressed raw honey

Rice cakes may look like polystyrene packing material but with a tasty spread can make a delicious and nutritious meal. Spread thinly with butter or non-hydrogenated vegetable margarine and best quality honey. Again, you'll find the right ingredients in your health-food store.

V *Hunza Apricots with Yoghurt*

7 or 8 Hunza apricots
1 medium carton of plain sheep's yoghurt

Hunza apricots can be purchased in dried form from the health-food store. To prepare, rinse them thoroughly, place in a small bowl and cover with filtered water. By morning you will have dark, sweet and tender apricots. Discard the stones (not difficult) and serve the apricots with the yoghurt for a deliciously nutritious breakfast.

This is an excellent combination for anyone who has a tendency to irritable bowel syndrome or constipation.

V *Scrambled Eggs with Vine Tomatoes*

2 large free-range eggs
1 tablespoon of filtered water
1 tablespoon of single cream
1 teaspoon of extra virgin olive oil
Sea salt and black pepper to season
2 vine tomatoes

Beat the eggs, water, and cream together until well mixed.

Wipe the inside of the pan with the olive oil.

Place the pan on a medium heat.

Add the egg mixture, stirring all the time.

Once or twice during cooking — and immediately before serving — flick the eggs gently around the pan with a hand whisk. This removes any lumps and makes the mixture light and fluffy.

Add sea salt and black pepper to taste.

Grill the vine tomatoes to accompany.

Scrambled Eggs and Smoked Salmon

This is one of my favourite breakfasts when I'm away on book or lecture tours. A meal sustaining enough to carry me through to lunch time. The recipe is a million miles away from the ghastly *just warm egg with a piece of salmon thrown on the side* that sometimes shows up on the worst of hotel breakfast menus.

You may wonder why anything containing eggs, cream, *and* butter together could possibly be helpful to anyone wanting to lose weight but, because the ingredients are so filling, this one course is enough and you probably won't want anything else until the middle of the day.

A good knob of butter (about 1 level teaspoon)
2 large free-range eggs
1 tablespoon of filtered water
1 tablespoon of whipping or double cream
2 slices of smoked salmon, chopped up into tiny pieces
Sea salt and black pepper to season

Melt the butter in a pan.

In a large bowl, whisk the eggs with the water and the seasoning.

In another bowl, whisk the cream until it's fluffy but not too stiff.

Pour the egg mixture into the pan, stirring constantly.

Just as you can feel the eggs beginning to set (but before they are fully cooked), remove the pan and whisk the mixture once or twice – nothing more than a couple of flicks of the wrist, really.

Return to the heat and stir in the smoked salmon and the cream. Another minute should make sure that the salmon is heated through. Serve immediately.

From the weight and the energy point of view, this breakfast will be digested more efficiently if you forgo the toast or any other starch accompaniment.

If you're short of time, throw the cream, eggs, water, and seasoning in the pan all at once, stirring madly. Add the salmon at the end as before. The result will be good but not so fluffy!

Undyed Smoked Haddock with Poached Egg

1 fillet of undyed smoked haddock
1 large free-range egg

You will need a small pan or egg poacher for the egg and a deep fry pan or skillet for the fish.

Place the cleaned fish in one pan and cover with cold filtered water. Place over the heat and bring the water to the boil.

Next, take the egg pan and fill with water. To save time, use water that you have just boiled in the kettle. Add the egg. If you are using an egg poacher, oil the poaching cup with a little butter or olive oil to prevent sticking. Keep an eye on both pans. Once the fish water has boiled, the haddock should take about the same time to cook as the egg. Lift the fish carefully using a fish slice. Place the egg, sunny side up, on top of the fish.

TEN

Quick and easy lunches and simple suppers

࿎

V *Cheese Omelette with Onion and Herbs*

2 large free-range eggs
1 tablespoon of filtered water
1 dessertspoon of extra virgin olive oil
1 organic onion (finely chopped)
1 teaspoon freshly chopped herbs (parley, thyme, basil, and
coriander all taste good with eggs)
Sea salt and black pepper to season

Heat the oil in a suitable pan and add the onion. Sauté until tender.

Beat the eggs and the water until the mixture is an even colour. The omelette will have a fluffier finish if you use an electric whisk.

Pour the mixture over the onion. Sprinkle with the herbs and a little seasoning. Cook until almost set.

Fold in half and continue cooking for a further 1 minute. Serve with Green Salad (see page 170).

V *Avocado and Hummus Salad*

1 avocado
1 small tub of prepared hummus
Good serving of Mixed Salad (see pages 169–70)

Prepare the Mixed Salad.

Cut the avocado in half, remove the stone and fill the hollow with hummus. Sprinkle with black pepper. Serve with the salad.

> Unless you are preparing this lunch for two, save money and time by keeping the other half of the avocado and the rest of the hummus for tomorrow's lunch. Run a little fresh lemon juice over the cut half of the avocado, turn it upside down on a plate, cover and seal the plate with cling wrap and place in the salad drawer of the refrigerator.

V *Chunky Vegetable Soup*

This is a wonderfully sustaining and warming soup which provides more than a full ration of the recommended daily vegetable intake. The quantity here is enough for two portions. Any remainder can be refrigerated overnight or popped into the freezer.

2 leeks or 2 organic onions

2 courgettes

1 head of broccoli

1 turnip

2 organic potatoes

2 organic carrots

1 dessertspoon of extra virgin olive oil

Filtered water or vegetable stock

1 teaspoon freshly chopped chives

1 dessertspoon of spirulina flakes

Seasoning as required

Wash and chop all the vegetables into small chunks. Discard the outer skin of each leek, cut the leek nearly in half lengthways and open it up under a cold running tap to remove all traces of grit or soil. Wash and chop all the vegetables into small chunks. Wash but don't peel the potatoes or carrots.

Heat the oil in a large pan. Add the vegetables and turn them over in the hot oil for 2 minutes.

Then add enough filtered water or stock to cover the vegetables.

Bring to the boil and then turn down to simmer.

Add the chives, cover, and leave to simmer until the vegetables are tender. (A sharp knife should slide through a piece of carrot with ease but not break it in half.)

Remove the pan from the heat and allow to cool. (If you need the soup straight away, there is no need to wait until the vegetables are cold, just cooled enough to liquidize safely.)

Place all ingredients in the blender including the fluid (you might need to do this in two batches) and turn on for 5 to 10 seconds only. If you like a smoother soup, blend for longer. Alternatively, hand blend in the pan, or use a potato masher.

Just before serving, stir in the spirulina flakes.

Serve piping hot with pitta, naan bread, or rye crackers.

Vitamin Tip: If you are cooking vegetables at any time (say, with an evening meal) and have any water left over that you can't use, keep it to add to soup recipes. Although not all the nutrients will be retained, it should stay fresh in the fridge for 24 hours if covered.

V *Artichoke Soup with Nutmeg and Parmesan*

8 to 10 Jerusalem artichokes
1 organic onion
1 dessertspoon extra virgin olive oil
2 good pinches of nutmeg
Filtered water or vegetable stock
1 tablespoon of freshly grated parmesan

Wash and chop the artichokes and onion. Sauté in olive oil for 2 minutes.

Add the nutmeg and stir it in.

Cover the mixture with filtered water and cook until the artichokes are tender.

Cool sufficiently to liquidize safely. Blend for 20 to 30 seconds or until completely smooth.

Return to the pan, add the parmesan and reheat until the cheese has just melted.

Serve at once.

If you want to keep any of this soup for use next day, put in it an airtight container in the refrigerator once it has cooled and add the cheese when you reheat.

V *Thick and Creamy Lentil and Potato Soup*

1 cup of red lentils
½ teaspoon of butter
2 shallots
4 large organic potatoes
Filtered water or vegetable stock
1 tablespoon single cream
Sea salt and black pepper to taste
1 dessertspoon of spirulina (optional)

Soak the lentils in filtered water overnight.

Next day, melt the butter in a suitable pan.

Wash and chop the shallots and sauté them in the butter for 2 to 3 minutes.

Wash and chop the potatoes into small chunks, leaving the skins on.

Strain the lentils, discarding the soaking water. Add the lentils to the pan and cover with 2 pints of fresh filtered water or stock. Simmer for 30 minutes.

Add the potatoes to the pan and stir round several times. Cook until the potatoes are tender (approximately another 10–15 minutes), and then remove from the heat.

Liquidize until smooth. Reheat, and just before serving stir in the cream and the seasoning, and sprinkle on the spirulina.

Serve with Matzo crackers or rice cakes, spread with a little butter.

V *Colourful Veggi Casserole*

2 medium organic potatoes

6 baby corns

4 cherry tomatoes

6 small button mushrooms

1 organic carrot

1 courgette

1 small red bell pepper (capsicum)

1 shallot or small onion

1 clove of garlic

1 tablespoon of extra virgin olive oil

1 teaspoon of ready-made mustard

A good pinch of mixed herbs

1 dessertspoon of potato flour

1 pint vegetable stock

Wash all the ingredients thoroughly.

Put the potatoes to one side.

Leave the corns, cherry tomatoes, and mushrooms whole.

Chop the carrot, courgette, and pepper into similar bite-size pieces.

Chop the shallot and crush the garlic.

Heat the oil in a large pan and sweat the shallot and the garlic for 2 minutes.

Stir in the mustard and herbs.

Next, add all the remaining vegetables except the potatoes.

Turn gently for about 5 minutes.

Tip the contents of the pan into a large oven casserole dish.

Stir in the flour so that all the ingredients are coated.

Slice the potatoes (leave the skins on if they are organic) and lay the slices over the other vegetables so that the dish is capped.

Pour the vegetable stock over and put on the lid.

Cook at 150° (300°F / Gas mark 2) for 2½ hours, removing the lid for the last 30 minutes of cooking time.

If you have no fresh vegetable stock available, dissolve a vegetable stock cube or heaped teaspoon of stock paste in a pint of boiling water. Health-food stores sell a good range of additive-free, yeast-free vegetable stock in cube, powder, and paste form.

V Jacket Potato with Choice of Fillings

There is nothing so comforting on a cold, wet or stressful day as a piping hot jacket spud. The best tasting jackets are done in a conventional oven although most restaurants and take-aways microwave for speed and convenience. If you have an oven timer at home that you can rely on, why not prepare jacket potatoes so that they are ready to eat when you get in. This is the best method I have found.

Choose your potatoes carefully, picking the best possible quality – organic if possible so that you can really enjoy eating the skins.

Wash them thoroughly, removing any eyes. Stab them evenly seven or eight times with a skewer. Place them on the rack in a hot oven (200°C / 400°F / Gas mark 6) for about 90 minutes. If the oven is on a timer, wrap each potato in cooking foil to help prevent shrinkage if you are delayed in taking them out of the oven.

If wrapped in foil and then in newspaper after cooking, jackets will keep hot for at least an hour, usually two, without further cooking.

Here are ten filling ideas, all of them vegetarian:

1 Hummus
2 Baked beans
3 Coleslaw
4 Aubergine dip (most supermarkets stock ready-made dips)
5 Mushrooms (chop them and fry them in extra virgin olive oil)
6 Leeks in white sauce (chop the leeks into tiny pieces and cook in filtered water until tender; make a basic white sauce with the cooking water and a little single cream)
7 Mozzarella
8 Vegetarian pâté
9 Grated Salad Garnish (page 171)
10 Parsley butter (a teaspoon of very finely chopped parsley blended into 1oz (30g) of softened butter

V *Wholemeal Pitta Bread with Choice of Fillings*

1 or 2 wholemeal pitta breads
Butter, non-hydrogenated vegetable margarine, or, for a very
healthy alternative spread, use mashed avocado

Here are ten filling ideas, all of them vegetarian:

Cold:
- Avocado and tomato
- Avocado and crisps – health-food stores have a range of healthier crisps
- Beansprout and beetroot (see below)
- Green Salad (page 170)
- Hummus
- Coleslaw

Hot:
- Baked beans
- Fried mushrooms
- Sauté potatoes (see Hearty and Healthy Chip Butties on page 158)
- Grilled tomatoes

Beansprout and Beetroot Pittas:
To fill 2 pitta breads, you will need a handful of beansprouts, about 6 thin slices of beetroot (3 for each pitta), and plain mayonnaise. This is a deliciously different filling but can be messy so it's not recommended for travelling – or for eating or preparing without a bib!

Use either beetroot that has been cooked from fresh and pickled at home or bottled beetroot in red wine or cider vinegar. Shrinkwrapped pre-cooked beets are not nearly as tasty, in addition to which they contain preservative.

One quarter avocado is usually enough for 2 large pittas. Save the rest by coating with lemon juice (see page 143), covering and refrigerating until next day to use with salad or jacket potato.

V *Quick Can Salad*

1 small can of sardines or salmon (in water or brine)
Large portion of Summer or Winter Salad (pages 169 and 170)

Although tinned food is generally regarded as being less nutritious than fresh equivalents, canned sardines and salmon are valuable for their magnesium, iron, and those all-important essential fatty acids (see Chapter 6). They are also one of the very best sources of calcium. Keep a can or two in the cupboard for emergencies. Tinned tuna is another nutritious reserve but not nearly so rich in calcium because the bones are not used.

V *Mixed Vegetable Mozzarella*

This makes an easy and light vegetable meal on its own or can be added as a vegetable dish to other ingredients for a more substantial main course.

1 small head of broccoli/calabrese
2 organic carrots
1 leek
1 courgette
4oz (110g) mozzarella cheese, sliced

Wash all the vegetables thoroughly and chop them into small chunks/florets. The broccoli stalk is rich in calcium so, if it's tender (cuts easily and doesn't look stringy), cut it into thin slices and include it with the florets.

Steam the vegetables until just cooked.

Drain well. Tip them all into a shallow oven dish. Sprinkle over a few drops of soy sauce. Spread the cheese over the top and grill until golden.

V *Sultana Rice and Beans (Serves 2)*

This recipe makes two ample portions. Any remainder will refrigerate well until next day if covered well. However, cooked rice should not be kept for more than 24 hours.

> 2 teaspoons balsamic vinegar
> 2 teaspoons extra virgin olive oil
> A touch of black pepper and sea salt
> 4 cups of cooked brown rice
> 1 can (200g) sweetcorn niblets
> 1 can (200g) mixed pulses
> 2 tablespoons of cooked garden peas
> 2 tablespoons of organic sultanas

To make the dressing, shake the vinegar, oil and seasoning in a jar until well mixed.

Place all the ingredients except the dressing into a large bowl and stir until the colours are evenly distributed.

Sprinkle the dressing over and mix again.

Serve this lunch on its own or with a Green Salad (page 170).

Use any leftovers for Avocado and Rice Tortillas (page 160) tomorrow or as part of Rainbow Rice (page 156).

V *Easy Leek and Potato Soup*

For two generous portions, you will need:

4 small or 3 large leeks
6 (egg-sized) organic potatoes
Filtered water
1 teaspoon of potassium salt
1 teaspoon of mixed mustard
2 teaspoons single cream
1 teaspoon finely chopped parsley (optional)

Wash and chop the leeks and potatoes (leave the skins on) and cook in filtered water until tender.

Cool sufficiently to liquidize safely. Add the salt, mustard, and cream and blend for 20 to 30 seconds. Reheat gently; don't allow to boil.

Sprinkle with chopped parsley and serve piping hot with warmed ciabatta bread or rice cakes.

V *Cheese and Tomato Crumpet*

This could be called a pauper's pizza. It's certainly delicious and much quicker to make.

2 crumpets
1 dessertspoon of your favourite chutney (I use a tomato and garlic pickle)
2 thin slices of mozzarella cheese
2 skinned tomatoes
4 black olives (stoned and halved) to garnish

Toast the crumpets on both sides.

Spread the top side of each crumpet with the chutney. Cover with the mozzarella.

Slice the tomatoes as thinly as you can. Lay them over the cheese. Garnish each crumpet with 4 olive halves.

Place them under a hot grill until the cheese starts to sizzle. Don't put them too close to the heat, otherwise the tomatoes will burn before the cheese is melted.

> Skin the tomatoes by placing them in a heat-proof jug and pouring boiling water on to them. After 30 seconds (no longer), pour the water away and you'll find that the skins lift off the tomatoes with ease.

V *Matzo Crackers with Tomato and Avocado*

4 Matzo crackers
½ avocado
2 skinned tomatoes
Sea salt and black pepper to taste

Spread each cracker with avocado and cover with slices of skinned tomato (see above). Sprinkle with salt and black pepper.

V *Crudités with Curd Cheese*

For speed and convenience, you can buy crudités ready prepared at most supermarket counters. It is also usually cheaper to make your own, especially if the left-over ingredients (you are unlikely to use a whole head of celery at one meal, for example) are used for the next day's salad or soup. Quantities will depend on you! Preparing 'to order' means that the vegetables will retain more nourishment.

Celery

Organic carrot

Baby tomatoes

Red bell pepper (capsicum)

Curd cheese (for dip)

Wash all the vegetables, including the tomatoes, really thoroughly. Cut the required amounts of celery, carrot, and pepper into strips. Arrange them on a plate with the tomatoes and the cheese.

Wrap the remaining vegetables carefully and put them in the salad drawer of the refrigerator.

V *Crudité Soup or Salad*

Chop the vegetables left over from yesterday's crudité. Either cook and liquidize them into soup or add them to the basic Green Salad (page 170).

Prawn and Pepper Quick-Fry

1 multipack of mangetout, baby carrots, and baby corns

1 small pack of cooked prawns

¼ each of red, green and yellow pepper

4 small organic mushrooms

1 small organic onion

1 teaspoon of ready-mixed mustard

½ teaspoon of cumin powder

2 teaspoons of balsamic vinegar

1 tablespoon extra virgin olive oil

Wash the carrots, mangetout, and corns. Trim if required. Cook them for 3 minutes either in a very little water or a steamer. Rinse in cold water and set aside.

Slice the onion, peppers, and mushrooms into strips and fry in the olive oil until the onion is clear.

Stir in the mustard and cumin and cook for a further 2 minutes.

Add the prawns and the cooked vegetables.

Stir thoroughly over the heat until all the ingredients are heated thoroughly.

Just before serving, mix in the balsamic vinegar.

Serve with a Green Salad (page 170).

V *Pasta Robusto*

8oz (225g) fusilli (pasta twists)

Filtered water

3 tablespoons extra virgin olive oil

2 medium organic potatoes cut into small chunks

1 small onion

½ red pepper

1 teaspoon mild curry powder

1 teaspoon chopped fresh basil (if available) or ¼ teaspoon Italian Seasoning

4oz (110g) chopped sun-dried tomatoes

Cook the fusilli in filtered water according to the pack instructions. Remember that some types (rice twists for example) will cook very quickly. (A knob of butter added to the cooking water will help to stop the pasta boiling over.) Once the pasta is cooked, drain it using a large sieve, rinse with cold water, and put to one side.

Heat 2 tablespoons of the olive oil in a large frying-pan. Fry the potato chunks in the oil, turning frequently until they are well browned.

Heat the remaining 1 tablespoon of olive oil in a separate

pan. Chop the onion and pepper into very small pieces and fry them until tender. Add the curry powder, herbs, and the sun-dried tomatoes. Simmer for a further 5 minutes.

Tip the onion and pepper mixture and the pasta into the pan with the potatoes. Stir until all the ingredients are heated through.

Top with Grated Salad Garnish (page 171).

V *Rainbow Rice*

Some of the ingredients for this recipe are similar to those in the Sultana Rice and Beans lunch dish (page 151) but the taste is quite different.

4 cups of cooked brown rice
1 small can (200g) of sweetcorn
1 can (200g) of mixed pulses
2 tablespoons of cooked petit pois
A tablespoon of chopped sun-dried tomatoes
½ red pepper (chopped into the tiniest pieces)
A good pinch of paprika
1 tablespoon of your favourite mayonnaise

Place all ingredients into a large bowl and stir until everything is distributed evenly. Serve hot or cold in pittas, naan bread, or with Green Salad (page 170).

V *Vegetarian Minestrone with Penne*

I make this soup using a deep-sided frying-pan but any large pan will do as long as it has a wide base and well-fitting lid. The soup is so chunky that it is almost a meal by itself. This quantity makes two good portions. If you can't imagine minestrone without parmesan, then add a sprinkling before serving.

2 small or 1 large tomato
1 onion
1 stick of celery
1 organic carrot
1 leek
1 courgette
1 tablespoon of chopped sun-dried tomatoes
1 clove of garlic (optional)
1 tablespoon of extra virgin olive oil
Sea salt and black pepper
Pinch of paprika
1oz (30g) penne pasta
Filtered water
1 pint of vegetable stock

Wash all the vegetables thoroughly.

Skin the tomatoes (see page 153).

Slice the onion into thin strips. Chop the celery, carrot, leek, courgette, and skinned tomato into small chunks. Slice the sun-dried tomato into tiny slivers.

Crush the garlic.

Fry the onion and the garlic in the olive oil for a couple of minutes.

Add all the other vegetables, paprika, and seasoning. Stir and turn them and then leave them to cook for a further 5 minutes.

In a separate pan, add the pasta to salted boiling filtered water and cook for 5 minutes.

Make a quick vegetable stock using an organic stock concentrate such as Plantaforce. (Health-food stores usually have a good range.)

Add the pasta and the stock to the vegetables, cover the pan and leave to simmer for about half an hour (20 minutes will be enough if you chop the vegetables into even smaller pieces).

Once cooked, test the soup for seasoning and adjust accordingly.

Serve on its own or with Matzos.

V *Hearty and Healthy Chip Butties*

For two substantial portions, you will need:

4 medium potatoes
Sea salt or salt substitute
2 tablespoons of extra virgin olive oil
4 brown pitta breads
Any fresh lettuce

This is one of the most satisfying, comforting snacks ever. Quick to prepare, and extremely nourishing, warming and filling. Buy organic potatoes (old or new will do). All supermarkets stock them. Leave the skins on. Wash well, and scrub out any eyes and green parts. In a flat skillet or frying-pan, heat the olive oil until hot but not smoking hot. Slice the potatoes into small scallop shapes. The size will depend upon the original size of each potato but you should be aiming for a quarter of an inch (½cm) thickness and approximately two inch (5cm) squares or rounds. Slide the potato slices into the oil and cook until brown and just beginning to crisp. Shake the pan during cooking to prevent sticking. Then turn each slice over and cook the other side in the same way. Total cooking time is usually about ten minutes. Just before you take the potatoes out of the pan, sprinkle them with salt and shake them around. Then tip them into warmed pitta breads and top with crispy lettuce.

For extra flavour, add sliced skinned vine tomatoes and a little mayonnaise or drop of French dressing.

> This recipe is dedicated to Eddie Blower at Beer Davis Publicity, my driver on the super successful *Food Combining Diet* book tour who voted my chip butties 'the best ever'. They're healthier without the tomato ketchup, Eddie!

V *Potato Chip Tortillas*

Instead of filling a pitta bread with the sauté potatoes (as in Hearty and Healthy Chip Butties), simply use two corn tortillas for each 'butty'. Tortillas are now available from all major supermarkets and some delis and bakeries, and they make a nice change from bread. Heating tortillas is quick and easy. Packs carry full instructions and other recipes.

V *Speedy Gonsalsa*

This is a mild variation of chilli hot salsa with a 'MexItalian' flavour.

1 organic onion
¼ each of red, green and yellow pepper
1 crushed garlic clove
1 tablespoon of extra virgin olive oil
4 vine tomatoes
¼ teaspoon cumin
Pinch of sea salt
1 teaspoon red pesto (the best quality pesto is made with extra virgin olive oil)

¼ teaspoon mixed herbs
1 teaspoon cider vinegar
2 corn tortillas

Slice the onion and the pepper and fry them with the crushed garlic in olive oil for 2 minutes.

Skin (page 153) and chop the tomatoes and add them to the pan, together with the cumin, salt, pesto, herbs, and cider vinegar. Simmer for 10 minutes.

Fill 2 hot corn tortillas with the mixture and top with Grated Salad Garnish (page 171). Alternatively, use the Salsa and Garnish as toppings for plain pasta twists or brown rice.

V Avocado and Rice Tortillas

For two good portions:

1 medium ripe avocado pear
Sea salt and black pepper to season
6 corn tortillas
1 tablespoon of extra virgin olive oil
Any leftovers from yesterday's Sultana Rice and Beans (page 151)

Mash the avocado with the seasoning.

Warm the tortillas according to the pack instructions.

Heat the oil in a suitable pan and fry the rice mixture.

Remove the tortillas from the oven and 'butter' each inside surface with the mashed avocado.

Fill with the hot rice mixture and serve immediately.

V Simple Pasta with Pesto

For this, the quickest and most popular of suppers, choose

the colourful rice pasta twists or delicious rice and ginseng twists from the health-food store. They cook quickly and are wheat- and gluten-free.

> 2–3oz (55–85 grams) of pasta
> Filtered water
> A knob of butter
> 1 tablespoon of green pesto sauce

Bring a pan of salted filtered water to a rolling boil. Add the butter and, once it has melted, add the pasta. Cooking time varies depending upon the type of pasta chosen, so check the pack instructions before you begin. Some kinds, especially rice pastas, will turn to 'porridge' if left too long.

Once cooked, drain through a sieve, return the pasta to the pan, and stir in the pesto.

Serve with any of the salads on pages 169–72.

V *Sugar Snap Stir-fry*

Here is another quick idea to save you time and satisfy your appetite. Choose the quantity of vegetables according to how hungry you are. Any leftovers can be refrigerated overnight to make a great next-day salad with a favourite dressing.

> 1 serving of sugar snap peas
> 1 serving of baby corns
> 1 serving of baby carrots
> 1 serving of young asparagus shoots (if available)
> 1 small onion (finely sliced)
> 1 clove of garlic (crushed)
> Filtered water

When choosing your pesto, fresh is always best. However, keeping
qualities are not great (a few days at most). If you are busy, have
little time for shopping, and if, like me, you use a lot of different
pasta recipes, it's worth buying a jar of really top-quality pesto that
has a longer life. Pick one made with extra virgin olive oil. Always
replace the cap securely after use and keep in the refrigerator once
opened.

1 tablespoon of extra virgin olive oil
1 serving of capsicums (any colour, cut into thin strips)
1 good pinch of mixed herbs
Sea salt and black pepper to season
1 teaspoon of ginger (for real bite, crush a piece of fresh ginger
about the size of a garlic clove; otherwise, use ½ teaspoon of
ground ginger)

You will need a wok or frying-pan and an ordinary saucepan.

Wash and trim the sugar snaps, corns, carrots, and
asparagus and cook them in boiling filtered water for 2
minutes.

In the frying-pan or wok, sweat the onion and the garlic
in the olive oil for 2 minutes.

Strain the vegetables and add them, together with the
strips of capsicum, herbs, salt, black pepper, and ginger, and
stir-fry the whole lot for a further 5 minutes.

Serve the stir-fry with brown rice.

V *Creamy Cabbage Casserole*

This makes a nutritious accompaniment to other dishes but
also a filling snack on its own.

1 small green cabbage with a good heart
1 small organic onion
2 medium organic potatoes
Black pepper
½ pint of vegetable stock
Half a small carton of single cream (about 2fl. oz/60ml)

Wash the cabbage and cut into slices. If bits of it fall apart, don't worry, just add them along with the rest. Peel and slice the onion. Scrub and slice the potatoes, leaving the skins on.

Layer all the ingredients into a large oven casserole. Start with a layer of cabbage, then onion and finally a layer of potato. Sprinkle with black pepper. Add the vegetable stock. Then pour the cream over the potato top and put the lid on to the casserole dish.

Place the dish into a medium oven (180°C/350°F/Gas mark 4) for 2 hours.

V *Buckwheat Noodles with Cabbage (Serves 2)*

This recipe gives you the opportunity to use up any spare cabbage and potato from the Creamy Cabbage Casserole (see above). It is wheat-free and gluten-free.

1 dessertspoon extra virgin olive oil
Filtered water
4oz (110g) buckwheat noodles (health-food stores or delicatessens should be able to order this for you if they don't already hold it in stock – if you can't get hold of these, try buckwheat fusilli or rice noodles instead)
4oz (110g) green cabbage, shredded finely
4oz (110g) organic potatoes, in small pieces

2oz (55g) butter

1 clove of fresh garlic, crushed

2 teaspoons finely chopped parsley .

1 teaspoon finely chopped sage

A sprinkling of ground nutmeg

4oz (110g) freshly grated parmesan

Add the olive oil to a large pan of boiling filtered water. Drop in the noodles, cabbage and potato and cook for about 10 minutes or until all ingredients are tender.

While the cabbage, noodles, and potato are cooking, melt the butter in a frying-pan and add the garlic, parsley, and sage, cooking gently for only about 1 minute.

Drain the noodle mixture and spread evenly over a warmed serving dish. Pour on the garlic and herb butter and mix in gently.

Sprinkle with the nutmeg and the parmesan.

Serve at once or, if the dish has lost a little of its temperature, pop under a hot grill for 1 minute.

V *Vegetarian Bolognese*

1 organic onion, sliced roughly chopped

1 clove fresh garlic, crushed

1 tablespoon extra virgin olive oil

2 tomatoes, finely chopped

½ red pepper, finely chopped

1 good pinch of mixed herbs

1 small pack of Quorn mince

1 tablespoon of tomato purée

2 tablespoons of red wine

¼ pint (125ml) vegetable stock

Filtered water

3–4oz (85–110g) spaghetti (or use legume pasta which is wheat-
free and gluten-free)

Sweat the onion and the garlic in the olive oil for 2–3 minutes.

Add the chopped tomatoes, red pepper, and herbs.

Add the Quorn and fry for a further 5 minutes or until the
Quorn begins to brown.

Then stir in the tomato purée and red wine. Add vegetable
stock until the mixture is just 'fluid' but not runny or watery.
Leave to simmer.

Meanwhile, bring a panful of salted filtered water to a
rolling boil.

Add the spaghetti or legume pasta. Cook as per pack
instructions.

Pour the Quorn mixture over the pasta and serve immediately with one of the salads on pages 169–72.

Quorn mince is a useful protein for those who don't eat meat.
However, it can be bland and needs the support of herbs and spices.

V *Spicy Vegetable Casserole with Brown Rice*

This dish is mildly spicy. If you like a more powerful punch,
double up on the cumin, coriander, and curry powder.

1 organic onion
1 clove of fresh garlic, crushed
1 tablespoon extra virgin olive oil
½ teaspoon cumin
½ teaspoon mild curry powder
½ teaspoon dried coriander
½ teaspoon ground ginger
1 teaspoon tomato purée

1 small head of cauliflower
1 small head of broccoli
2 organic carrots
1 leek
½ green pepper
8 organic button mushrooms
1 dessertspoon potato flour
8 cherry tomatoes (skinned – page 153)
1 pint (570ml) of vegetable stock
2 dessertspoons of frozen or fresh peas

In a large skillet or frying-pan, sweat the onion and garlic in the olive oil for a couple of minutes.

Stir in the cumin, curry powder, coriander, ginger, and tomato purée.

Leave to cook for a further 2 minutes.

Break the cauliflower and broccoli into baby florets. Prepare all the other vegetables and chop them into bite-size pieces, keeping the tomatoes separate. Chop the carrots and leeks into small chunks.

Add the cauliflower, broccoli, carrots, leek, green pepper, and mushrooms to the frying-pan. Stir round for a further 5 minutes. When everything is well coated with the onion and spices, tip the contents into a large oven dish with a well-fitting lid. Then stir in the potato flour. Add the fresh tomatoes and the stock.

Place in the oven at 150°C (300°F/Gas mark 2) for 90 minutes.

Then remove the casserole and stir in the peas. Put back into the oven for a further 30 minutes.

Serve with brown rice.

Any leftovers can be refrigerated and reheated thoroughly for next-day use.

V *Egg-fried Rice*

1 small organic onion
1 large flat mushroom
1 tablespoon of extra virgin olive oil
Half a small red capsicum (red pepper)
A pinch of paprika
A pinch of hot curry powder
A pinch of mixed dried herbs
2 cups of cooked brown rice
1 tablespoon of cooked petit pois
A good sprinkling of soy sauce
2 free-range eggs, hard boiled and chopped
Dark green lettuce leaves finely shredded

Slice the onion and the mushroom and fry in the olive oil for 2 minutes. Shell the eggs and cut them into small pieces.

Wash and deseed the red pepper and chop into tiny fragments.

Add the pepper to the pan along with the paprika, curry powder, and herbs and cook for a further 1 minute.

Then toss in the rice, the peas, and the soy sauce and heat through thoroughly.

Just before serving, mix in the chopped egg.

Tip the whole lot out on to a bed of lettuce.

Bean Bake

Quick, convenient, filling and nourishing. Because of the size of the cans, it is very difficult to make just one single portion. This lot makes two good servings. Delicious (and colourful) served with sugar snap peas, mangetout, or petit pois.

2oz (50g) fusilli pasta twists – cooked
Filtered water
1 tablespoon of extra virgin olive oil
1 clove of fresh garlic, chopped
1 organic onion, chopped
½ teaspoon fresh rosemary leaves
1 organic carrot, grated
1 small can of red kidney beans
1 small can of chickpeas ⎫ or 1 large can of mixed pulses
1 small can of butter beans ⎭
1 small can of sweetcorn kernels
1 dessertspoon of Molkosan whey (page 172)
1 tablespoon of pumpkin seeds
Sea salt and black pepper

Cook the pasta in the normal way in filtered water.

In a separate, deep-sided frying-pan, heat the oil and sauté the garlic, onion, and rosemary gently for 2 minutes. Then add the carrot, beans, and sweetcorn. Stir together and cook for a further 5 minutes.

Add the cooked pasta. Stir in the Molkosan whey. Sprinkle the pumpkin seeds over. Add seasoning if required. Serve at once.

V Mixed Vegetable Gratin (Serves 2)

This is the simplest, quickest, and easiest of all vegetable dishes. Ready in a trice, nourishing, and filling.

1 small head of cauliflower
1 small head of broccoli
1 leek
1 turnip

1 parsnip
Sea salt and black pepper
4 thin slices of mozzarella cheese
A good sprinkling of ground nutmeg

Wash and prepare the vegetables, chopping them or breaking them into evenly sized smallish pieces.

Steam them until just tender. Drain off any excess water and tip the vegetables into an ovenproof dish. Sprinkle with black pepper and sea salt. Lay the cheese over the vegetables. Sprinkle on the nutmeg. Pop the dish under a hot grill until the cheese melts and bubbles.

Serve straight away.

Super salads

To accompany main courses or to eat on their own. Try to include as many of the ingredients listed here as are available. Make up as much as you think you need, depending upon whether the salad is a light meal on its own or accompanying a main course.

V *Mixed Summer Salad*

Any dark leaf lettuce
Rocket
Favourite fresh herbs
Vine tomatoes (skinned)
Slices of avocado
Watercress
Red, green, or yellow bell pepper
Beansprouts
Sunflower seeds
Pumpkin seeds

SIMPLE DRESSING:
2 teaspoons organic cider vinegar
1 teaspoon of extra virgin olive oil
Black pepper and sea salt to taste

Prepare the salad and sprinkle with the seeds. Mix the vinegar, oil, and seasoning and add to the salad.

V *Mixed Winter Salad*

Shredded red cabbage
Any dark leaf lettuce
Grated carrot
Mustard and cress
Celery
Chicory
Grated raw beetroot or beetroot in red wine
Spanish onion (optional)
Seedless raisins
Pine nuts

SIMPLE DRESSING:
Balsamic vinegar
Extra virgin olive oil
Black pepper
Celery salt

V *Green Salad*

Watercress
Any dark leaf lettuce
Dandelion leaves
Rocket
Young spinach leaves

Any fresh herbs; for example, parsley, chives, mint, marjoram,
coriander, or green basil

V *Grated Salad Garnish*

This is a wonderful topping for almost any meal you care to
mention and so quick to prepare. Particularly tasty on pasta
and rice dishes. Also goes down well with people who would
otherwise not eat salad or vegetable foods. This lot makes
enough for four. If you need less, it's best to use half a carrot,
half an onion, etc., and to wrap and refrigerate the unused
portions for use next day. Once chopped or grated, most
foods lose a lot of their vitamin content.

1 organic carrot
1 small mild onion or, if not available, use salad onions
1 small white radish or a few ordinary red radishes if white is not
available
A stick of celery
1 pepper (red, yellow, or green)
A chunk of crisp lettuce or cabbage
Soy sauce, cider vinegar, herb salt, and black pepper to taste

Wash the ingredients thoroughly and peel them, removing
any tough bits, stalks, etc. Grate the whole lot so that it is as
finely shredded as possible. Mix in a shake of soy sauce, a
tablespoon of cider vinegar, and seasoning to taste. Add as
much of the salad as you like to top off your pasta or other
dishes.

V *Tomato Salad*

2 medium tomatoes per person, skinned and sliced
4 fresh basil leaves, finely chopped

2 teaspoons of extra virgin olive oil
1 teaspoon of balsamic vinegar
A good twist of black pepper

Lay the prepared tomatoes in a shallow dish (a small china flan dish is about the right shape and size).

In a jar, shake the basil, balsamic vinegar, olive oil, and black pepper.

Pour the mixture over the tomatoes.

For a sharper bite, an unusual alternative to any salad vinegar is Bioforce Molkosan, a lacto-fermented whey which is particularly beneficial to the digestive system. Molkosan is also valuable as a drink first thing in the morning (see also Molkosan Punch on page 184). See Chapter 12 for supplier information.

V *Avocado and Asparagus Salad*

The only ingredients you will need are:

Asparagus spears
1 green pepper (capsicum)
1 ripe avocado
Any dark green lettuce
Sea salt and black pepper

Trim and cook the asparagus in boiling water until just tender.

Cover, cool, and refrigerate.

Slice the pepper into very fine strips. Slice the avocado. Cover a dinner plate with shredded lettuce leaves. Lay all the pepper, avocado, and asparagus on to the leaves. Season the plate with the sea salt and black pepper.

ELEVEN

Easy entertaining

ॐ

In this section you will find a dozen delicious dinners, giving you plenty of entertaining choices during your new healthy eating plan. There are five vegetarian options plus two fish, one seafood, one red meat, and three poultry dishes. All meals serve two. Just increase the quantities if you have more guests or halve them if you are having a special dinner alone.

For the red meat and poultry meals, seek out a supplier of organic farm produce. (Chapter 12 has details.)

Main courses

Garlic Chicken Breast

Anyone who can't – or chooses not to – eat garlic can substitute a good strong mustard, mixing it with the butter as described.

Don't forget to use organic free-range poultry if possible.

2 organic free-range chicken breasts
2 cloves of fresh garlic, crushed (or 1 teaspoon of strong mustard)
Sea salt and black pepper
1oz (30g) soft (salted) butter
1 tablespoon of extra virgin olive oil

Split each chicken breast lengthways with a sharp knife. Mix the crushed garlic (or mustard) with the butter and spread half into each portion of chicken.

Heat the olive oil in a frying-pan, and add the chicken.

Cook gently for 10 minutes each side. Season just before serving.

Serve with any fresh vegetables or one of the salads on pages 169–72.

Big Heap Tiger Prawn

Buy as many peeled tiger prawns as you think you can eat comfortably without feeling over-full; ten per person is usually about right.

Make the Sugar Snap Stir-fry (page 161) but without the brown rice. Add the prawns to the pan along with the vegetables and 2 tablespoons of white wine.

King prawns are a good substitute if tiger prawns aren't available.

Lamb's Liver in Red Wine Gravy

Not suitable, of course, for vegetarians but an excellent source of a whole range of nutrients including Vitamin A and iron. Choose enough lamb's liver so that there are four or five thin slices per serving.

2oz (50g) of butter
2 tablespoons of extra virgin olive oil
1 small organic onion, very finely chopped
Lamb's liver (quantity as above)
1 dessertspoon buckwheat flour
4 tablespoons of red wine
Vegetable stock
Sea salt and black pepper

Melt the butter and olive oil in a frying-pan. Sweat the onion until clear. Add the liver, cook for no more than 2 or 3 minutes, turning once.

Remove from the pan and put to one side.

To make the gravy, add the flour to the juices, oil and onion remaining in the pan and stir to a paste. Add the wine, and then the vegetable stock a tablespoon at a time, stirring constantly, until you have a thick gravy.

Return the liver to the pan for a couple of minutes to heat through.

Season and serve at once with any choice of fresh vegetables.

Scrambled Eggs and Smoked Salmon

This delicious breakfast dish also makes a terrific dinner, especially when served with a fresh green salad or fresh spinach. And it's so satisfying that you're unlikely to want starters or puddings. See page 140 for the recipe, but double-up the quantities.

Serve with the Green Salad (page 170) or freshly steamed young spinach leaves.

Turkey Breast with Mustard Sauce

Find a supplier of organic meat and poultry (see Chapter 12 for details).

1 teaspoon of any favourite grain mustard
1oz (25g) soft (salted) butter
1 tablespoon of extra virgin olive oil
4 flat mushrooms, chopped very finely
Sea salt and black pepper
2 turkey breasts

Split each piece of turkey lengthways with a sharp knife.

Mix the mustard with the butter and spread half into each turkey breast.

Heat the olive oil in a frying-pan, add the mushrooms, and cook for 1 minute, turning them all the time.

Then add the turkey.

Cook for 10 minutes each side. Season just before serving.

Serve with any fresh vegetables or one of the salads on pages 169–72.

Honey Roast Chicken with Chives

1 organic free-range chicken (choose a size depending on how many mouths you are feeding)
1 tablespoon of cold-pressed raw honey
A good handful of fresh chives, chopped up very finely

Wipe the chicken (you won't need the giblets) and rub the outside surface with the honey. Then sprinkle on the chives so that they stick. Wrap the chicken in foil and place it upside down in a roasting dish and pop into a hot oven. The cooking time will depend on the size of bird.

Half way through the cooking time, turn the chicken the right way up. This method makes for much juicier breast meat.

If you don't have chives, or can't buy them, a tasty alternative is to rub the surface skin with half an onion *before* spreading the honey. Then push the onion inside the chicken.

V *Cauliflower Casserole*

1 leek

1 medium-size cauliflower (choose one with nice white flesh and
crispy green leaves)

1lb (450g) Jerusalem artichokes (use a mixture of swede
and parsnip if artichoke is out of season)

Filtered water

Sea salt and black pepper

2 shallots

1 tablespoon of extra virgin olive oil

1 dessertspoon of potato flour

1 tablespoon of single cream

1 small pack of goat's cheese

A sprinkling of nutmeg

Wash and chop the leek and cauliflower. Tear the green leaves
from the outer stalks of the cauliflower and shred them up like
lettuce. If the stalks seem tender, chop them too. Discard anything tough or stringy. Cook the leeks and cauliflower
together, saving any water from the boiling or steaming.

Scrub the artichokes and, in a second pan of filtered water,
boil them until tender. When cooked, mash the artichokes
with a potato masher, adding the sea salt and black pepper.

Meanwhile, chop the shallots and fry them in the olive oil.
Add the flour to make a paste and then, adding the saved
vegetable water a drop at a time, make the sauce.

Next, take an open oven dish. Tip the cauliflower and
leeks into it. Spread the mashed artichokes over the top. Pour
the cream over the artichokes and then the sauce over everything so that the vegetables are covered. Dot the whole lot
with blobs of goat's cheese. Sprinkle with nutmeg. Pop
under a hot grill for a couple of minutes so that the cheese is

just melting and all the ingredients are piping hot.
Serve with buttered carrots and green peas.

V *Pasta with Peppers and Peas*

Filtered water
1 knob of butter (about ½ teaspoon)
A shake of soy sauce
½lb (225g) penne (short hollow tubes of pasta)
1 clove of fresh garlic, crushed
1 tablespoon of extra virgin olive oil
1 heaped tablespoon of green pesto sauce
1fl. oz (28ml) of vegetable stock
1 tablespoon of frozen petit pois
½ red pepper, deseeded and shredded very thinly

Bring a pan of salted filtered water to a rolling boil. Drop the
butter and the soy sauce into the water. Add the pasta and
cook until just tender. Drain off the water and return the
pasta to the pan.

In a frying-pan, sauté the garlic in the olive oil for 1 minute.

Stir in the pesto sauce and then the vegetable stock. When
well mixed, add the petit pois and red peppers and cook until
the pepper is just softened (about 5 minutes).

Then pour the pesto mixture over the pasta. Stir well and
serve with Tomato Salad (page 171).

If you used goat's cheese yesterday and have any left over,
dot the salad with small pieces of this.

V *Hot Rice and Snow Pea Salad*

2 cups of cooked brown rice
2 portions of snow peas (mangetout)

2 shallots, or 1 onion
½ green pepper
A good handful of rocket
A good handful of lamb's lettuce
A generous pinch of dried mixed herbs
1 dessertspoon of extra virgin olive oil
1 dessertspoon of pumpkin seeds

Cook the brown rice.

Wash and trim the snow peas. Chop the shallots (or onion) and the green pepper into the tiniest pieces. Shred the rocket and the lamb's lettuce and lay them on to a dinner plate.

Fry the shallots (or onion) and the pepper with the herbs in the olive oil for 2 minutes. Then add the snow peas and cook for a further 2 minutes. Finally, throw in the rice and pumpkin seeds and keep the whole lot moving for a minute or so until everything is hot through.

Tip the contents on to the green leaves. Serve immediately.

Rolled Lemon Sole in White Wine Sauce

2 fillets of lemon sole, skinned and rolled up
1 cup of dry white wine
1oz (30g) butter
1 dessertspoon of flour (for thickening)
1 dessertspoon single cream
Grated parmesan to garnish

Poach the rolled fish in the white wine.

As soon as the fish is cooked (a sharp knife should pass right through the centre of each roll without resistance) lift it out of the pan into a shallow grill dish.

In a basin (or pestle and mortar) mix the butter and the flour to a smooth paste. Drop the mixture and then the cream into the remaining wine, stirring continuously. When the sauce has thickened, pour it over the fish. Sprinkle with grated parmesan and pop under a hot grill for about 60 seconds.

Serve with freshly cooked spinach.

V *Fusilli with Sage and Sun-dried Tomatoes*

Enough fusilli for two
Filtered water
1 tablespoon of red pesto sauce
1 tablespoon of chopped sun-dried tomatoes
1 tablespoon of pine nuts
2 fresh tomatoes, cut into small wedges
1 teaspoon of finely chopped sage

Cook the fusilli pasta as per pack instructions, in filtered water. Then stir everything else into the pasta and serve at once. This meal is delightful served as a cold lunch.

V *Pinwheel Pasta with Pepper and Pine Nuts*

Enough rotelle (pinwheel pasta) for two (choose a pack containing red, green, and white pasta)
Filtered water
1 spoonful of vegetable stock powder or paste
1 fresh garlic clove, crushed
1 small piece of fresh ginger, crushed
1 shallot, chopped
1 dessertspoon of extra virgin olive oil
8 to 10 baby button mushrooms

A handful of sliced green beans (any kind will do as long as they are
young and tender)

½ red pepper, chopped into very small pieces

1 tablespoon of pine nuts

Bring a pan of filtered water to a rolling boil. Add the vegetable stock and, once dissolved, add the pasta and cook it in
the usual way.

Meanwhile, in a large frying-pan, sauté the garlic, ginger,
and shallot in the olive oil. Throw in the mushrooms and green
beans and cook for a further 3 or 4 minutes; then add the
pepper pieces and continue cooking for a further 2 minutes.

Drain the pasta and tip it into the other ingredients. Mix
together, sprinkle on the pine nuts, and serve with any of the
salads from pages 169–72.

Sweet treats

V *Fresh Fruit Fool*

Any 2 pieces of ripe fruit, e.g. kiwi, peach, nectarine, mango, pear,
or banana

1 tablespoon of double cream

2 tablespoons of sheep's yoghurt

1 teaspoon of cold-pressed liquid honey

1 teaspoon of sweet wine or sherry

2 teaspoons of flaked almonds

Wash and peel the fruit and chop into smallish pieces.

Put into a liquidizer with the cream, yoghurt, honey, and
alcohol and blend until smooth.

Serve in sundae glasses and sprinkle the top with flaked
almonds.

V *Crunchy Crumble*

2 large cooking apples
  (sliced) and
1 cup of fresh blackberries

} or {

If fresh fruit is not available use:

1 can of apricots in natural juice
1 can of pears in natural juice
1 can of blackberries in natural
  juice

For the crumble topping:

2oz (55g) desiccated coconut
2oz (55g) grounds almonds
1oz (30g) pumpkin seeds
1oz (30g) sunflower seeds
1oz (30g) oat bran
1oz (30g) best quality brown sugar
2oz (55g) butter

Wash, peel and slice the apple very thinly and layer it into a pie dish. Wash the blackberries and tip them over the apple. If you have no time for preparation, use the canned fruit suggested above (minus the juice).

For the topping, take all the ingredients (except the butter and sugar) and grind them in a suitable blender or coffee grinder until you reach the 'fine breadcrumb' stage.

Stir in the brown sugar. Mix in the butter, either by hand or machine.

Tip the mixture on to the fruit and bake in a medium oven for 10–15 minutes.

Serve with a little cream or yoghurt.

V *Melon and Grape Salad*

½ ripe melon
A handful of seedless grapes
2 sprigs of mint

Scoop out the melon flesh into a dessert dish or sundae glass with a teaspoon or melon scoop. Cut the grapes in half, and pile them on top of the melon. Garnish with the mint.

> Melon skin in particular harbours the germs that cause serious food poisoning, so it is especially important to follow the rule of washing all fruit before preparing or serving.

V *Honey Yoghurt*

1 medium carton of sheep's yoghurt
1 teaspoon of cold-pressed liquid honey

Simply stir the honey into the yoghurt and enjoy!

Suitable for anyone with a cow's milk allergy or intolerance, this delicious mixture makes the ready-prepared honey yoghurts taste very ordinary.

V *Banana Cream Yoghurt*

1 medium carton of sheep's yoghurt
1 banana (not too green, not too ripe)
1 teaspoon of dark molasses sugar

Mix all the ingredients together in a blender.

Serve immediately, otherwise the banana will turn brown.

V *Organic Chocolate*

Most people enjoy a chunk or two of chocolate at the end of an entertaining evening meal. Most supermarkets now stock organic chocolate which tastes absolutely delicious. See Chapter 12 for more information.

V *Molkosan Punch (Serves 6)*

1 fresh ripe mango
1 small fresh ripe melon (any kind, but galia or canteloupe are best)
2 fresh ripe kiwi fruit
1 bottle of Bioforce Molkosan
17fl. oz (500ml) red grape juice (choose non-carbonated)
17fl. oz (500ml) organic apple juice (choose non-carbonated)
Juice of 1 lemon

Juice the mango, melon and one of the kiwi fruits through your juicing machine. Stir into a punch bowl with the Molkosan, grape, apple, and lemon juices. Peel and slice the other kiwi fruit and float the slices in the punch for decoration.

Makes 6 double servings.

If fresh mango and melon are not available, look for a bottled tropical juice mix in your local health-food store or delicatessen.

PART FIVE

Resources

TWELVE

Where to find ...

৵

Suppliers

Biocare
Mega EPA 1000mg Fish
Oil capsules
Mega GLA
Magnesium Ascorbate
Vitamin C
Enzyme-Activated
B Complex
Adult One-Daily Vitamins
and Minerals
(contains B vitamins)
Bio-acidophilus
Garcinia cambogia

Biocare Ltd, Lakeside, 180
Lifford Lane, Kings Norton,
Birmingham B30 3NT.
Telephone: 0121 433 3727

Bioforce
Bambu coffee
Herbamare sea salt with
herbs
Trocamare sea salt with
spices
Plantaforce vegetable
bouillon organic stock paste
Alpamare soy sauce and
vegetable seasoning
Molkosan lacto-fermented
whey
Also a wide range of herbal
tinctures

Bioforce, Olympic Business
Park, Dundonald, Ayrshire
KA2 9BE. Telephone:
01563 851177

Blackmores
Fish oil 1000mg
Bio-C Low Acid formula
vitamin C complex
Executive Formula B (also
contains vitamin C)
Ginkgo biloba

Acidophilus and Bifidus
Organic Spirulina Crystal
Flakes

House of Blackmores, 37
Rothschild Road, Chiswick,
London W4 5HT.
Telephone: 0181 987 8640

Kordel Uk
Ginkgo biloba

Kordel UK, York House,
York Street, Bradford,
Yorkshire BD8 0HR.
Telephone: 01274 488511

Pharma Nord
Bio-Quinone (co-enzyme
Q10)
Bio-Antioxidant (contains B
vitamins)
Bio-Marine Fish Oil capsules
Bio-C Vitamin
Bio-Biloba (Ginkgo biloba)
Bio-Glandin (GLA)

Pharma Nord UK Ltd,
Spital Hall, Mitford,
Morpeth, Northumberland
NE61 3PN. Telephone:
0800 591756 or 01670
519989

Solgar
A wide range of vitamin,
mineral and herbal
products, available at most
health stores.

Solgar Vitamins, Aldbury,
Tring, Herts HP23 5PT.
For stockists' details
telephone: 01442 890355

Xynergy Health Products
Aloe 99
Aloe Vera Gel
Lifestream Aloe Vera
Biogenic Juice
Organic Spirulina

Xynergy Health Products,
Ash House, Stedham,
Midhurst, West Sussex
GU29 0PT. Telephone:
01730 813642

Special foods

**Free-range and organic
meat, poultry, and
vegetables**
For details of stockists in
your area contact The Soil
Association, 86 Colston

Street, Bristol, Avon BS1 5BB. Telephone: 0117 929 0661

Cold-pressed raw organic honey
New Zealand Natural Food Company, Unit 7, 55–57 Park Royal Road, London NW10 7JP. Telephone: 0181 961 4410

Green & Blacks organic chocolate
Telephone: 0171 243 0562 for stockist information.

Specialist foods for those on wheat-free and gluten-free diets
Virani Food Products Ltd, 10–14 Stewarts Road, Finedon Road Industrial Estate, Wellingborough, Northamptonshire NN8 4RJ. Telephone 01933 276483

Kjaess Food for Life, 56E Upper Montagu Street, London W1H 1FP.
Telephone their helpline 0171 723 0091 for stockists

of gluten-free, dairy-free, yeast-free and sugar-free foods. Kjaess foods are already available in some of the major supermarkets.

Tests available for nutritional deficiencies, food allergies, etc.
Biolab, 9 Weymouth Street, London W1N 3FF.
Telephone: 0171 636 5905/5959

Tests also available to qualified practitioners
Biocare, Lakeside, 180 Lifford Lane, Kings Norton, Birmingham B30 3NT.
Telephone: 0121 433 3727

Practitioners

The following multi-therapy centres are staffed by qualified practitioners, offering a wide range of services and information.

All Hallows House, Idol Lane, London EC3R 5DD. Telephone: 0171 283 8908 (Monday to Thursday)

If you are outside London, All Hallows will try to help you find a practitioner nearer to your home. To obtain the *All Hallows Foundation Practical Guide to Candida*, send a cheque for £8.25 to Green Library, 6 Rickett Street, London SW6 1RU.

The Alternative Health Information Bureau, 2 Upper Station Road, Radlett, Hertfordshire WD7 8BX. Telephone: 01923 469495

The Bureau holds information on alternative therapies and a database of research material is available at modest cost to practitioners and the general public. They also publish a bi-monthly journal. If you are looking for a qualified practitioner, AHIB can put you in touch with relevant associations.

The Hale Clinic, 7 Park Crescent, London W1N 3HE. Telephone: 0171 631 0156.

The House of Blackmores, 37 Rothschild Road, Chiswick, London W4 5HT. Telephone: 0181 987 8640

THIRTEEN

References

᠁

Can diet products help you slim? *The Food Magazine*. July/September 1991, pp14–15. The Food Commission.

Anderson, O. Endurance and exercise. *Peak Performance*. June 1994;45:1–3.

Genetic engineering breeds costly protest. *Washington Post* (Federal page). 17 November 1994.

Guyton, A. C., Digestion and absorption in the gastrointestinal tract. *Textbook of Medical Physiology*, W. B. Saunders, 1991, pp726–9.

New weight-loss drug far from a miracle. *Tufts University Diet and Nutrition Letter*. June 1996;14[4]:6.

Report on artificial sweeteners. *The Food Magazine*. July/September 1996;34:6–8.

Stricter weight guidelines in the offing. *Tufts University Diet and Nutrition Letter*. September 1995;13[7]:3–6.

The Slimming Scandal, *The Food Magazine*, February/April 1992 pp8–9. The Food Commission.

Theories on yo-yo dieting unwind. *Tufts University Diet and Nutrition Letter*. December 1994;12[10]:1–2.

Toubro, S., and Astrup, A., Randomised comparison of diets for maintaining obese subjects' weight after major weight loss: ad lib, low fat, high carbohydrate diet v. fixed energy intake. *British Medical Journal* 1997; 314: 29–34.

Treadmills make best indoor calorie burners. *Tufts University Diet and Nutrition Letter*. June 1996;14[4]:1.

Women's Environmental Network. Pesticides in chocolate. *The Food Magazine*. October/December 1995;31:5.

Working Party on Pesticide Residues. Report on lindane in milk supply. *The Food Magazine*. July/September 1996;34:1.

FOURTEEN

Further reading

❧

First class guides to the treatment of candidiasis
The Practical Guide To Candida by Jane McWhirter (The All Hallows Foundation/Green Library)
Beat Candida by Gill Jacobs (Vermilion)

The original easy-to-follow best-sellers on healthy eating and safe, sensible dieting
Food Combining In 30 Days by Kathryn Marsden (Thorsons)
The Food Combining Diet by Kathryn Marsden (Thorsons)

Essential reading for anyone who cares about the real quality of food and the way food is produced
The Food We Eat by Joanna Blythman (Michael Joseph)
Very highly recommended.
Fats That Heal, Fats That Kill by Dr Udo Erasmus (Alive Books)
Additives – Your Complete Survival Guide by Felicity Lawrence (Century)
Food Adulteration and How To Beat It from The London Food Commission (Unwin)
Fast Food Facts by Tim Lobstein (Camden Press)

On relationships and personal growth
Men Are From Mars, Women Are From Venus by Dr John

Gray (Hodder & Stoughton)
   Mars And Venus In The Bedroom by Dr John Gray (Hodder
& Stoughton)
   The Joy of Sex Pillow Books by Alex Comfort (Mitchell
Beazley)
   Emotional Intelligence by Daniel Goleman (Bloomsbury)

More recipe ideas – superb but simple
   Leith's Cooking for One or Two by Caroline Waldegrave
(Bloomsbury)
   Leith's Healthy Eating by Puff Fairclough, Anne Heughan
and Caroline Waldegrave (Bloomsbury)
   Soups by Marguerite Patten (Bloomsbury)

FIFTEEN

Reader information

∽

The information that Kathryn includes in her books, feature articles, and lectures has been accumulated from her own personal research, training, and experience which, from the feedback she has received, would appear to have helped many people. However, it is important that the reader understands that these guidelines are not intended to be prescriptive, nor are they an attempt to diagnose or treat any specific condition.

If you are concerned in any way about your health, Kathryn recommends that you visit your own doctor or hospital consultant without delay. She also suggests that you keep your medical adviser informed of any dietary changes and of any supplement programmes you intend to follow. Obtain as many details about your condition as possible, asking plenty of questions about any medicines that may be prescribed to you. Do not stop taking any currently prescribed medication without first talking to your general practitioner.

Follow a varied and sensible diet that contains plenty of fresh unprocessed wholefoods and daily fresh fruits and vegetables. Take regular exercise and avoid cigarette smoke.

Kathryn regrets that, due to the cost and time involved in dealing with her already overloaded mailbag, she can no longer reply individually to letters or comment on specific case histories. She is, however, always delighted to hear from readers and promises to read every letter.

SIXTEEN

Index of recipes

ج

Vegetarian options are marked **V**